Everyday

Healing

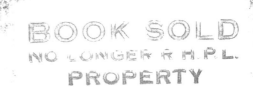

EVERYDAY
Healing

Stand Up, Take Charge, and Get Your Health Back...
One Day at a Time

》《

Janette Hillis-Jaffe

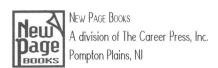

New Page Books
A division of The Career Press, Inc.
Pompton Plains, NJ

EVERYDAY HEALING
EDITED BY ROGER SHEETY
TYPESET BY EILEEN MUNSON
Cover design by Joanna Williams
Printed in the U.S.A.

To order this title, please call toll-free 1-800-CAREER-1 (NJ and Canada: 201-848-0310) to order using VISA or MasterCard, or for further information on books from Career Press.

CAREER
PRESS

New Page BOOKS

The Career Press, Inc.
12 Parish Drive
Wayne, NJ 07470
www.careerpress.com
www.newpagebooks.com

Library of Congress Cataloging-in-Publication Data

Hillis-Jaffe, Janette, 1969-

Everyday healing : stand up, take charge, and get your health back... one day at a time / by Janette Hillis-Jaffe.

pages cm

Includes bibliographical references and index.

ISBN 978-1-60163-370-5 (paperback) -- ISBN 978-1-60163-382-8 (ebook) 1. Health--Popular works. 2. Nutrition--Psychological aspects--Popular works. 3. Food habits--Psychological aspects--Popular works. 4. Self-care, Health--Popular works. I. Title.

RA776.H58 2015

613.2--dc23

2015008946

》《

For my mother,

Jane Hillis,

and in memory of my father,

Jim Hillis.

Thank you for everything.

》《

»»»»»» Acknowledgments ««««««

I would never have been able to write this book if I hadn't first gotten healthy enough to do so. I want to thank the many people who shepherded me on my path to wellness and contributed much of the wisdom shared in this book. I deeply appreciate the dozens of healthcare providers I saw and particularly want to thank Ilana Margalit; Dr. Tracy MacNab; Jill Swyers; Dr. Heidi Fleiss-Lawrence of the Jerusalem Family Wellness Center; Peg Baim and the staff at the Benson Henry Institute for Mind Body Medicine at Massachusetts General Hospital; Dr. Alex Bingham and Dr. Glenn Rothfeld at the Rothfeld Center for Integrative Medicine in Waltham, Massachusetts; and Brian and Anna Maria Clement and the entire staff at the Hippocrates Health Institute in West Palm Beach, Florida.

Thank you also to the angels who helped run our house for years when I was too sick to do any of it: Sacha Mackerweicz, Yasmina Kamal, Daniella Mendola, Pramn Sansuwan, and especially Alison Montillo. Much love and gratitude to Ariel, Sabrina, Yaakov, Ness, Yovel, and Menachem Burger for providing a second home to my husband and sons when I needed space to rest during the hardest times. Special love and thanks go to my teacher Jaye and listening partners Mark, Sasha, and Ilana. Their consistent caring and support when I could barely leave the house for years helped make everything possible.

It is still a miracle to me that this book is written and out in the world. I am grateful to so many people for making it a reality. I want to thank my agent, John Willet from Literary Services, Inc., a gem of a man who believed in this project, gave it its title and format, and searched tirelessly for a publisher. A heartfelt thank you goes to Michael Pye and everybody at New Page Books for taking a chance on a new author. Beth Lieberman's brilliant editing gave the book shape and order. Rich Klin fine-tuned the final product. Author's coach Ann McIndoo helped me give the book its first form. I could not have written it or gotten it published without the encouragement and wisdom of Steve Harrison and the whole gang at Bradley Associates and the Quantum Leap program.

A special thanks goes to my friend and author Marilyn Paul, who said I should write a book in the first place and gave me constant encouragement and advice. The time and talents of Mary-Liz Murray, Alexis Lefort, and Sandy Spector have all been critical in developing and sharing my ideas. Tovah Lazaroff's assistance in gathering and writing healing stories was an enormous help. I deeply appreciate my friends and family who provided valuable feedback on early teleseminars and book drafts: Ronit Ziv-Kreger, David Ziv-Kreger, Ziesl Maayan, Michal Oshman, Ariel Burger, Ellen Krause-Grosman, Kevin Wrathall, Donna Trader, Beth Jaffe, Djana Paper, Ilana Margalit, Sara Levine, Jennifer Weinstock, Ketriellah Goldfeder, Tsila Stone, Malka Sima Pais, Nancy Norton, Abigail Rose, Nina Englander, Andrew Dovid Shiller, and Stephanie Anderson. I am constantly inspired by my coaching clients for their strength, intelligence, and perseverance; and am grateful to each of them for sharing their wisdom and stories with me.

The stories in this book are culled from conversations with dozens of patients and providers over several years. I am indebted to them for their time and knowledge. I particularly want to thank the people who gave their time to be interviewed specifically for this book: Ziesl Maayan, Marilyn Paul, Dan Neuffer, Debbie Wolfe, Pattie Hulquist, Simon Pimenta, and Christina Hardy.

I could not have gotten healthy nor written this book without my amazing family. My mother, Jane Hillis, and my parents-in-law, Liz and Alan Jaffe, provided love and support in countless ways that made both healing and writing possible. The love, encouragement, and wisdom I received from Jamie Hillis, Jon Hillis, Donna Trader, Rich Jaffe, Kerri Jaffe, Bob Jaffe, and Beth Jaffe inspired me and kept me going through the rough times. I want to thank my amazing sons, Tani and Binyamin Hillis-Jaffe for being consistent sources of both comic relief and patience, when I was sick and when I was writing. There aren't enough words to describe how thankful I am for my husband, David. His wisdom and generous, loving support are the foundations that made both my healing and this book possible. I am grateful every day that I get to share my life with him.

Lastly, I once heard a gospel singer answer the question of how she developed her voice by saying, "All glory goes to God." I couldn't agree more. I thank the Divine for the lessons I learned in my search for wellness and for any success I had in transmitting them through this book.

»»»»»» Contents ««««««

Introduction   15

Practice 1. Take Charge   27

Day 1: Get on the Fast Track to Better Health   28
Day 2: Reject Hopelessness   29
Day 3: Tell Yourself the Truth   31
Day 4: Jump In: Feel the Pain—Feel the Rewards   34
Day 5: Jump In: What if You Accepted Your Reality?   35
Day 6: Become a Badass   37
Day 7: Choose an Inspiring Destination   39
Day 8: Melissa's Story: Shoot for the Stars!   41
Day 9: Embrace Change   42
Day 10: Jump In: What's Stopping You?   44
Day 11: Be Action-Oriented   45
Day 12: Commit   47
Day 13: Jump In: How Committed Are You?   48
Day 14: Set Limits to Set You Free   50
Day 15: Make Your Choices Count   51
Day 16: Activate Your Body's Healing Powers   53
Day 17: Be the Boss of Your Healthcare Team   56
Day 18: Ziesl's Story: It Was Up to Me   57
Day 19: Be Curious   59
Day 20: Make Good Hires   62
Day 21: Binyamin's Story: Don't Be Afraid to Fire   64
        Your Doctor
Day 22: Make Meetings Productive   65
Day 23: Manage Your Information   68
Day 24: Put First Things First   71
Day 25: Jump In: What Are Your Big Rocks?   72

Practice 2. Nurture Your Heart   75

Day 26: How Emotions Matter   76

Day 27: When Feelings Rule Your Decisions   77

Day 28: Identify the Tough Emotions   79

Day 29: Use Your Neocortex   80

Day 30: Let it Out   81

Day 31: The Healing Benefits of Tears and Laughter   82

Day 32: Listening Partnerships: Not Your Average Conversation   85

Day 33: Let Structure Create Safety   86

Day 34: Practice Deep Listening   88

Day 35: Rachel's Story: Thinking My Way Through Breast Cancer   90

Day 36: Reach for the Joy   93

Day 37: Increase Your Joy   94

Day 38: Find Joy Through Connection   96

Day 39: Create a Life You Want to Show Up For   98

Day 40: Liza's Story: Choosing Joy   99

Practice 3. Believe   103

Day 41: Cultivate Your Inner Quarterback   104

Day 42: Understand the Placebo Effect   105

Day 43: Become a Wholehearted Optimist   107

Day 44: Christina's Story: Confidence in My Recovery   109

Day 45: Jump In: Choosing Optimism   111

Day 46: Surround Yourself With Positive People   112

Day 47: Integrate Useful Feedback   113

Day 48: Cultivate Trust   114

Day 49: Replace Negative Thoughts With Positive Ones   117

Day 50: Notice Your Inner Critic   118

Day 51: Kick the Negativity Habit   121

Day 52: Jump In: Flip Your Negative Thoughts   122

Day 53: Jump In: Fire Your Inner Critic   123

Day 54: Make Stress Work for You   124

Day 55: Choose Your Response to Stress   125

Day 56: De-Stress Your Life   127

Day 57: Jump In: Prioritize Your Life   128

Day 58: Discover the Relaxation Response   130

Day 59: Practice the Relaxation Response   131

Day 60: Imagine a Fabulous Future   133

Day 61: Jump In: Use Visualization to Turbo-Charge Your Healing   135

Day 62: Be the Awe-Inspiring Hero of Your Own Life   137

Day 63: Talk About the Hardest Thing   139

Day 64: Believing at the End of Life   141

Day 65: Kris Carr's Story: Accepting Fear and Embracing Joy   143

Practice 4. Connect   **145**

Day 66: Deepen Your Relationships to Deepen Your Healing   146

Day 67: Be a Leader—Ask for Help   147

Day 68: Do You Really Need Help to Heal?   148

Day 69: Notice That You Are Not Alone   150

Day 70: Get Out of Your Way   152

Day 71: Jump In: What's Getting in the Way of Getting Connected?   154

Day 72: See the Support Around You   155

Day 73: Choose a Primary Support Person   156

Day 74: Hold Hands When You Head Into the Health-Care System   160

Day 75: Outsource the Details   162

Day 76: Healing Is Expensive—Ask for Help   164

Day 77: Find a Role Model   166

Day 78: Getting Support to Recover From Cancer Treatment   169

Day 79: Getting Support to Lose Weight   170

Day 80: Jump In: What Support Could You Use to Heal?   171

Day 81: Four Steps to Ask for What You Need   173

Day 82: Step 1. Inflation—Pump Up Your Self-Worth   174

Day 83: Jump In: Inflation—Some Quick Reminders   175
    That You Are Worth It

Day 84: Step 2. Explanation—Don't Suffer Alone   176

Day 85: Jump In: Explanation—Tell Your Story   177

Day 86: Step 3. Education—Share Information   178

Day 87: Step 4. Invitation—Make the Ask   179

Day 88: Gift Your Loved Ones With You   181

Day 89: Jump In: Map Your Healing Support Team   183

Day 90: Jump In: Notice Your Deep Connections   184

Practice 5. Create Order   187

Day 91: How Can Order Help You Heal?   188

Day 92: Marilyn's Story: Know What's Important   190

Day 93: Organizing Is Holy, Healing Work   192

Day 94: Jump In: What's Your Relationship to Order?   193

Day 95: Debbie's Story: Embrace Home-Care as Self-Care   195

Day 96: Make Space for What Matters   197

Day 97: Set Up Your Space Like a Kindergarten   199
    Classroom

Day 98: Five Steps to Organizing Your Space to Help   201
    You Heal

Day 99: Create New Systems   203

Day 100: Renovate Your Routines   204

Resources   207

Notes   211

Index   217

About the Author   223

»»»»»» Introduction «««««««

The future depends on what we do in the present.

—Mahatma Gandhi

Things were pretty dark in January 2008. I was taking two bioidentical hormones, a steroid, an anti-asthma medication, and more than 50 herbal and vitamin pills. I had recently finished six months of high-dose antibiotic therapy and had tried just about every alternative healing approach and most of the healing diets in the known universe. Two doctors said that I had chronic Lyme disease. Others said I had chronic fatigue syndrome, Myalgic Encephalomyelitis, or an unknown autoimmune disorder. All I knew was that I had a chronic cough, aches all over my body, vertigo, and fatigue so intense that some days I could hardly make a fist. I cancelled lunch with friends for my 39th birthday because sitting up and socializing was more than I could manage. I had felt that way, more or less, for almost six years.

Fast-forward to one year later, January 2009, when I threw myself a 40th-birthday party for 50 guests and danced for hours. I was no longer on any medications at all. I was running three times a week and finally getting back to work. After six years spent mainly in bed or in doctors' offices, all this "normal" activity felt like a gift. It was so good to be back.

How did I get from 2008 to 2009? By completely taking charge of my health. I overcame my resistance to change, got lots of help, dove into a fierce search for a new treatment approach, and adopted a new, healing lifestyle.

After years of searching for someone to cure me, I realized that it was up to me; although physicians and alternative healers often have life-saving treatments and advice to share, in my case most didn't. After a long search, the lifestyle that brought me back to full health was built on a plant-based diet, several detoxifying practices, nurturing my emotional well-being, and lots of high-quality sleep and exercise.

But this is not a how-to book for adopting that lifestyle. There are many paths to health. If you are dealing with a serious health challenge, this book is designed to give you the tools and skills to find and commit to your unique healing path, whatever that might be.

It's Hard—Let's Make it Easier

Whether you have chronic pain or illness, allergies, cancer, excess weight, infertility, a nagging injury, or persistent fatigue, you have probably put a lot of thought and effort into improving your health. You may have tried many things already and have more ideas in store. Some variation of treatment, plus the trio of diet, sleep, and exercise, floats in most of our minds. Hmm…finding the right treatment, eating right, sleeping enough, and exercising regularly—it sounds pretty straightforward. So, why aren't we all just doing it?

We aren't doing it because it's actually harder than it sounds. The crippling fatigue, pain, or other symptoms that sometimes accompany serious health can make the simplest acts torturous. Even if you don't have significant symptoms, staying on top of everything it takes to get healthy can be an enormous task. A friend can recommend a treatment she read about, but she won't spend hours researching its efficacy. Your physical therapist may encourage you to walk every day for exercise, but he won't be there when having to stop and rest after only a few minutes triggers an overwhelming wave of grief. Your nutritionist can suggest you avoid sugar, but is she going to dive between you and your friend's birthday cake? I don't think so.

So, I want to tell you two things:

1. You can make it easier for yourself—immensely so.
2. Even when it is hard, you are worth it. And you can do it.

Five Practices That Can Change Your Life

Looking back on my journey and hundreds of hours of conversations with others who have radically improved their health, I saw a pattern. Those people had all integrated the following five practices into their lives. In this book, we are going to take 100 days to explore them, one at a time.

Practice 1. Take Charge: Accept the full reality of your health challenge and take full responsibility for addressing it. Make healing your top priority, including making lifestyle changes where necessary and taking control over your health research, records, and decisions.

Practice 2. Nurture Your Heart: Use tools both to reduce the fear and anxiety that can sabotage your healing work and to increase the joy and clarity that can support it.

Practice 3. Believe: Adopt a fiercely confident attitude about yourself, your life, and your ability to achieve your optimal health.

Practice 4. Connect: Build a strong support team and enrich all your relationships in the process.

Practice 5. Create Order: Use organizing principles to establish systems that support your healing work.

Each of this book's 100 daily entries includes:

> › A thought-provoking quotation.

> › A short essay or success story, concrete examples, medical research, or an action or writing exercise to explore that section's practice.

> › A suggested action step or question for further exploration.

Rather than tell you what food to eat, how to exercise, or which treatment to try, I recognize that you already know much of that and can figure out the rest with wise guidance. The tough part is taking action. Trying to recover from a significant illness, lose excess weight, heal an injury, or get chronic symptoms under control is a part- to full-time job. In addition to researching new treatments and navigating the healthcare system, you may need to deal with big emotions, a new diet, medical bills, or challenging physical rehabilitation. Managing all of that is not easy. I've been there. I know.

It was so hard for me that when the diet that ultimately led to my healing was suggested to me in the first year of my illness, my reaction was "Are you crazy? Who eats like that?" It was just not a viable option for me at the time. I had to spend five years preparing myself emotionally, physically, spiritually, and logistically to take on that major healing effort.

Everyone has their own path to health. For some, it involves getting into the right clinical trial or finding the right surgical intervention. Others need a new diet and exercise routine. Virtually everybody benefits from making significant changes in their attitude and sleeping, eating, and exercise habits.

I want you to find and commit to your unique path to health sooner than the five years it took me. This book is designed to help you cut through whatever is getting in the way.

I invite you to take the next 100 days to think about your health differently, get more support, embrace change, and open opportunities for physical and emotional healing that you never imagined. Together, we will explore how to do the following and more:

> Acknowledge your current reality and set inspiring goals for the future.

> Creatively research your treatment options.

> Communicate effectively with healthcare providers.

> Work through the tough emotions that can derail your healing work.

> Create confidence that you can meet your health goals.

> Reduce, embrace, or manage stress.

> Cut your isolation and reach out successfully to family and friends for support.

> Establish routines that promote regular exercise, healthy eating, and high-quality sleep.

> Organize your living spaces to promote healthier living.

By providing concrete daily actions, exploring some logistical fixes, and reflecting on the tougher emotional aspects of healing, we'll chart a path to make your healing work easier, less isolating, and more effective.

My Story

I received the wisdom in this book from dozens of authors, teachers, healthcare providers, and fellow patients during my six-year struggle to get healthy. It was all instrumental in enabling me to find my path to health.

I was pretty high-energy as a young person. In my late 20s, in addition to working full-time and going out with friends, I volunteered for a few organizations and trained for charity events, like a 260-mile bike ride and a half-marathon.

Introduction

That all changed in the fall of 2002, when I was 33 and pregnant with my second son. I got laid up with a flu-like illness. I was feverish, achy, coughing, exhausted, and weak, and couldn't function for weeks. Months after the fever passed, I still ached all over and was so weak that I could barely walk around the block. But I was in denial. I was a high-energy go-getter; I'd be fine. So I ignored how I felt and pressed on as best I could.

One summer day in 2003, when my second son was about three months old, in spite of being exhausted and achy, I took my sons to the zoo. As we looked at the animals, the baby was asleep in a snuggly on my chest and his two-year-old brother happily ran around. Suddenly, my exhaustion, which had seemed manageable, turned into a nauseating fatigue so intense that I almost fainted in front of the lions' cage. I got dizzy, as I often did in those days, sat down heavily on a bench, and began to sob. I was so weak; I had no idea how I was going to drive us home or even make it back to the parking lot. I don't remember how I made it home that day. What I do remember is that I realized then that I was not well enough to take care of my children by myself. And that was terrifying.

I spent the next five years looking for someone or something that could heal me, all the while trying to raise my sons with my husband and do part-time fund-raising work for nonprofits when I could. I saw two or three of every specialist: endocrinologists, rheumatologists, infectious-disease doctors, and more. I tried every conventional or alternative treatment under the sun: hormones, antibiotics, supplements, special diets, meditation, qigong, talk therapy, acupuncture, herbs—you name it. But no matter what I did, I felt basically the same: achy, dizzy, exhausted, and weak, often with a terrible cough on top. Every day was an effort just to get by.

Finally, in 2008 it all came to a head in a Manhattan doctor's office. My primary doctor in Boston thought I might have chronic Lyme disease and recommended that I see a Lyme specialist in New York.

At the appointment, the doctor confirmed the chronic Lyme diagnosis and prescribed a cocktail of three powerful drugs: an antibiotic, an anti-parasite, and an anti-malarial. He couldn't guarantee that this would heal me and said that I might have to stay on the drugs for years and that there would most definitely be significant side effects. That didn't sound good, but I was desperate.

Even though I wasn't sure chronic Lyme was the correct diagnosis, I immediately filled the prescriptions and got up early the next morning to take the drugs. I stood in my dark kitchen, looking at the bottles, and began to think about the many potential side effects. I thought about the people I knew with chronic Lyme who had been on similar drugs for years and were still suffering terribly. I thought about how the doctor couldn't guarantee anything or put me in touch with anybody who had completely healed with this regimen.

I was terrified that I would never get well; that I would never play tag with my sons, have a meaningful job, or make it to a family vacation. The fact was I didn't believe that these medications would work. I just didn't know what else to do.

I sat down on the floor and began to cry. I don't know how long I sat there, sobbing and praying for help, but by the end I had reached some clarity for the first time in months. I had been asking healthcare providers to heal me for years and, as well-intentioned as they were, it wasn't working. I had to stop looking for a magic pill or treatment. I was the one who had gotten sick. I was the one who had to heal myself.

I put the medications back and went to wake up my husband, David. I announced, "I'm not going to take the drugs. I'm going to do whatever it takes to find people who have healed totally from this illness and then do whatever it takes again to follow their lead and get healthy myself. It might be pretty intense and I am going to need your help and a lot of other people's as well. Are you in?" He was pretty groggy, because it was about five in the morning, but he managed to croak out, "I'm in."

After that, I dove into researching my symptoms and possible treatments with a new frenzy. I spent hours talking to patients and doctors again, this time with a laser focus on finding people who had fully recovered, and a fresh openness to trying new things. Within three months I found several people who had healed illnesses similar to mine through a challenging plant-based diet supplemented with vegetable juices and sprouts, a lot of exercise, and a whole new, more positive attitude. After six years of debilitating illness, I was willing to try anything. With lots of support from friends, family, and my primary physician, I took on that new lifestyle.

What was the result? As you read in the first paragraph of this book, I danced for hours at my 40th birthday in January 2009 with my friends and family, returned to work that year, and started living life to the fullest again. It was so good to be back.

That was my path to health. What will yours be?

How to Use This Book
Embrace "A Little Bit Is Also Good"

One great thing about life is that, in order to make a change, we only need progress, not perfection. Rabbi Nachman of Breslov, a spiritual leader in the early-19th-century Hasidic movement of Judaism, famously said, "A little bit is also good." We can bring about real change in our lives by making several small adjustments that collectively enable us to reach our goals.

Just like bricks in a wall are made more stable as each brick is laid in around them, every piece of progress in one of the five practices in this book strengthens all the other practices as well. For example, if you create a bit more order through new systems to manage your medical information, it becomes easier to take charge and advocate for yourself.

There are many tips and ideas for how to adopt each of the five practices in this book. Challenge yourself to go beyond your comfort zone, but don't try to do them all. You don't need to do everything or be perfect—and that's a good thing, because you can't. You get to do what works for you and chart your own path. That, you can do.

Actively Engage

There are suggested thought exercises or actions at the end of most of the 100 daily entries. Other entries are titled with *Jump In* and feature activities like writing exercises to explore your emotions and attitudes, or action steps to get support or begin a self-care practice.

There are also dozens of concrete examples of how people have used these practices to support their healing. Take time to explore what you could learn from these stories and how you could apply that to your own life. These healing stories have been gathered through years of personal interviews, coaching sessions, and informal conversations with patients in a variety of settings. They are all true accounts of actual experiences. In some cases, composites have been used or names and personal details have been changed to protect privacy.

Keep in mind the quote attributed to Confucius: "I hear and I forget. I see and I remember. I do and I understand." Just reading these exercises, stories, and questions may help you think more clearly about your health, but actively engaging with them will enable you to take action, reshape your life, and find your healing path sooner. Pick up a pen or put your fingers on the keyboard; talk to a friend about these ideas; and explore them further online or in books or videos. Dive in and make them yours.

Ideally, the best way to engage with this book is to read it all first without doing the exercises, just to get the main ideas. Then go back and read one entry each day, giving yourself the time to grapple with the stories, daily actions and exercises through journaling, conversation, prayer, or whatever works for you. By taking this approach, you can achieve some amazing shifts in your life in 100 days.

Grab a Journal and a Calendar

Devote a notebook, journal, or new file on your computer to use with this book. You can write in responses to the daily prompts, do all of the Jump In and planning exercises, keep a running list of things you'd like to try to support your healing, and record your thoughts and feelings about the whole process.

If you don't regularly use a calendar—either paper or digital—this would be a great time to get one. Recognizing that you are more likely to do something when you have planned when and how you will do it, many of the exercises and daily actions suggest that you choose a time to do an activity and put it in your calendar right then to make sure it happens. Having both your calendar and your journal with you whenever you read the book will enable you to get much more out of the experience.

Embrace Both Passion and Patience

Harriet Tubman once said, "Every great dream begins with a dreamer. Always remember, you have within you the strength, the patience, and the passion to reach for the stars to change the world."

I love that she included both the heat of passion and the coolness of patience, which can seem like polar opposites, but are both necessary to achieve big goals. After your diagnosis or injury or after the symptoms of your undiagnosable "syndrome" become unbearable, it will be your passion for life that moves you to action. Your passion is what will fuel your desire to heal and enable you to railroad anyone or anything that gets in your way.

Introduction

Whereas your passion propels you to action, your patience will enable you to bear the challenges and overcome setbacks. Patience doesn't mean passively sitting around and waiting for someone to tell you what to do. It takes an enormous amount of inner strength to be patient and persevere.

According to Alan Morinis, a leader in the Jewish character-development practice of *Mussar*, "The Hebrew term for patience is *savlanut*. It shares a linguistic root with *sevel*, which means 'suffering,' and *sabal*, which means 'a porter.' What could these three words possibly share in common? The answer is that being patient means bearing the burden of your own suffering. You tell yourself, I can bear the feelings...and, not crumpling under their weight, you are patient."[1] I would also add that you don't have to—and indeed, shouldn't—bear those feelings alone. Practices 2 and 4, Nurture Your Heart and Connect, have some suggestions of how to get support.

In other words, being patient means hanging in there when the going gets tough, which, as you already know, comes with the territory of having a major health challenge. If your first (or second or third or fourth) shot at a healing path does not give you the results you want, it will be both your passion for life and your enduring patience that bring you back to try again.

Accept the Healing Cycle

The need for the delicate dance between patience and passion becomes even clearer when we acknowledge that healing is usually a cyclical, rather than a linear process. That means you may sometimes feel like you are running in circles. But don't despair. It's a spiral. Those circles are usually taking you somewhere higher, even if it doesn't feel like it.

The healing cycle has four distinct stages. They are:

> **Research:** Exploring your treatment options, including lifestyle changes, and conventional and alternative or supplemental treatments.

> **Experimentation:** Committing to one set of treatments for a period of time and evaluating the results. *Experimentation* is not a comforting word, but the reality is that when your healthcare provider says, "This has a 50-percent (or even a 95-percent) chance of working," you and she are embarking on an experiment to see how a treatment works on your body. That is the

case every time we take a pill, receive a treatment, change our diet, go to a physical therapist, or try any new approach to healing.

> **Healing:** Sometimes, your body responds to the first experiment (or group of experiments) and you achieve your optimal health. If not, then, as hard as it is, you go back to the research stage and begin again with new, useful information.

> **Maintenance:** Our bodies always require care and attention, particularly for those of us who have had or still have a major health challenge. Figuring out how to maintain optimal health is a lifelong pursuit for everybody.

Depending on the health challenge, a person can go through this cycle and arrive at maintenance in just a few months. For others, it may take many years. For millions of people with a long-term condition like juvenile diabetes, Parkinson's disease, multiple sclerosis, autoimmune illnesses, or some cancers, exploring new ways to manage their health using something akin to this cycle can be an ongoing effort that waxes and wanes their whole lives. For people experiencing infertility or chronic digestive troubles, fatigue, or pain with no clear diagnosis, it can take several trips through this cycle to identify both the root problem and the best way to address it. It goes without saying that it can be particularly frightening to go through the cycle more than once when you are facing a potentially terminal illness. Use the tools in this book on nurturing your emotions, reducing stress, and getting support to help you persevere.

Be Open to Exploring the Spirit

God comes up occasionally in this book. I recognize that God is a rather fraught topic. It tends to inspire or offend everybody a little differently. You may love God-talk. You may be completely turned off by the very concept of God. You may be a spiritual person with strong ideas about the Divine, but a distaste for organized religion. Or you may be none of these.

Whatever your thoughts are on this complicated topic, I invite you to do the best you can to open up to the explorations of spirituality and healing in this book. Spiritual and religious teachings have some of the greatest wisdom on both healing and making meaning from suffering. That wisdom shows up in a few spots throughout this book. If you are uncomfortable with the idea of God, whenever you see that word, please substitute in your mind any words that work better for you. Some possibilities include: *All benevolent power in the universe*; *That which unites all living things*; *Good Orderly Direction*; *Goddess*; *Good*; or *Nature*. Enjoy the creativity and be open to where it takes you.

Grab a Friend

Practice 4, Connect, focuses on getting support for your laundry, family care, emotions, food preparation, and everything else that may impact your healing process. If possible, it is also great to get support in going through this book.

You can do this in a couple of ways. Invite a friend to read the book with you, setting aside regular times to discuss its ideas and update each other on your progress and challenges. You can also pull together a group of three or more and run an *Everyday Healing* Action Group that supports its members in finding a healing path and committing to it. It's easy and makes the book more fun and effective. To help you do either of these, these two tools are available to download for free at *www.EverydayHealingforYou.com/tools*:

> › *Facilitator's Guide for Everyday Healing Action Groups.*

> › *Guidelines for Everyday Healing Partnerships.*

The accountability and support you will gain by working through the book with a partner or a group will increase its impact in your life exponentially. If you can set this up for yourself, I highly recommend it.

Lastly, I also lead live *Everyday Healing* Webinars, teleseminars, and in-person workshops on a variety of topics. I try to keep them affordable, action-oriented, and even a little fun. You can check at *www.EverdayHealingforYou.com/programs* to see what is available.

Now, let's dive into the first practice, Take Charge.

Take Charge

It will never rain roses. When we want to have
more roses, we must plant more trees.
—George Eliot

Over the years, I have met countless amazing people who have healed from, or vastly improved their lives while living with, every health challenge imaginable.

Every one of them has something in common. They take complete responsibility for their well-being. Instead of asking others, "What can you do for me?" they ask themselves, "What can I do for myself?"

You are powerful beyond your wildest imagination, but being sick, overweight, or in pain can make that hard to believe. You may feel terrible and have a hard time doing the basic activities of daily life. Plus, most of us have been taught from childhood to look outside of ourselves for healing. Take the cherry-pink syrup for a headache. Take the orange-flavored stuff for a cough.

This practice, Take Charge, is about uncovering how powerful you can be in your own healing. It's about noticing how precious you are, setting ambitious goals, making more time for self-care, advocating for yourself, and exploring new options that could transform your life. I imagine you have done a lot of that already. And I know it can be hard. Let's explore together how to dig down, do even more, and achieve the kind of health you dream about.

Day 1
Get on the Fast Track to Better Health

You can have results or excuses, but you can't have both.

—Unknown

As I wrote in the Introduction, I was encouraged to try the plant-based and green-juice diet that was central to my healing in the first year of my illness. Only, I waited half a decade to try it, until I was so desperate that I felt I had no choice. I don't want that for you. I want you to find your path to health sooner.

Again, I am not recommending my healing diet for everybody (although more vegetables in some form are always a good thing). We all have our own unique path to health. The sooner that you fully take charge of and commit to your healing, the sooner you will find yours.

So, what does *take charge of your healing* really mean? It's when you:

› Educate yourself about your health challenge(s) and take time to research a variety of treatment options.

› Make regular time in your schedule for nurturing your body and soul with self-care practices like exercise, healthy eating, sufficient sleep, and meditation or prayer.

› Be willing to try new things and change your perception of yourself (for example, trade a self-perception as a night owl for an early riser).

› Know how precious you are and that you are worth all the resources it takes to heal.

› Stop looking for others to cure you.

› Get support to do all of the earlier suggestions, because it can feel impossible. I know.

That list can be overwhelming. So remember: A little bit is also good. Usually, the more you do, the better, but often even just one significant change can make an enormous difference.

Joshua was 40 years old and a retail store manager when he started experiencing terrible back pain. It came and went, but for years it often kept him home from work and family outings. He was gaining weight, getting depressed, and missing out on life. A few friends encouraged him to try yoga to address the pain, but he insisted that he was not the "yoga-type."

Finally, after four years of intermittent, debilitating pain, it became constant. He was unable to work and was told that major surgery was his best bet. Luckily, his surgeon required that he do several sessions of aggressive physical therapy before he had the surgery. Six sessions into a course of physical therapy, Joshua was experiencing significantly less pain and after 12 sessions he was almost entirely pain-free. What did this physical therapy consist of? A combination of strengthening exercises, yoga stretches, and yoga breathing.

Although Joshua previously insisted that he was not the "yoga-type," he now regularly does several minutes of yoga stretches and breathing to protect his back and address any recurring pain.

For him, taking charge of his healing didn't mean a radical life change, but it did mean letting go of some preconceived notions and looking at what he could do for himself. Once he was willing to do that, he experienced healing that he calls "miraculous."

It sounds great, but I know it's not that simple. Taking charge doesn't happen overnight. People usually go through a series of steps to get there. We'll explore them together in the next few weeks.

>»> *For Today* «<<
What would taking charge of your healing look like? What self-perceptions could you let go of? What new thing could you try? What help could you ask for?

)(

Day 2
Reject Hopelessness

It is for us to pray not for tasks equal to our powers, but for powers equal to our tasks.

—Helen Keller

Let's not disregard a difficult reality. Sometimes people take charge of their health to the best of their ability and still don't achieve the healing they want. In spite of their best efforts, they aren't able to get out of the wheelchair, stop the progress of their disease, or completely free themselves from pain. Having witnessed this among people I love, I know the heartbreak, grief, and hopelessness it can bring. I encourage you not to give in to that hopelessness.

Don't let that heartbreak stop you from going all out in your efforts to heal, because these things are also true:

It All Makes a Difference

The efforts made by the people who seem to "not succeed" still have a huge impact on their lives and those around them. For example, my friend Jaye lived for 13 years after her first supposedly terminal illness, kidney failure. She worked and lived a life full of music, close friends, and family for most of that time, despite coming up against recurrent infections and throat cancer. She mobilized a great deal of resources and support and committed all her energy to heal from each health challenge she faced. And, although she died of cancer in the end, her life was much longer and richer for all her efforts.

You Can Take Charge in Any Circumstances

If the time ever comes to accept a heartbreaking health result, you and those around you will be much better equipped to handle it with strength, courage, and connection if you have been in charge of your health, educating yourself, leading your family and friends, and nurturing your body and soul all along.

Most of Us Can Achieve Our Goals

Fortunately, most of us, most of the time, do not need to accept such unwanted conclusions. And anyone who does would surely encourage the rest of us to use all of the resources we can to confidently pursue our health goals and fully embrace life while we can. There are advances in medicine every day and medical research constantly confirms how our lifestyle choices vastly impact our health. We don't have total control over our health, but we have more power than we know.[1]

This month I invite you to exorcise your excuses, dismiss your disbelief, and dive into taking charge of your healing in a way you never have before. It could spare you years of suffering and get you to your new, healthier life much faster.

»»» *For Today* «««
Explore what disappointing health outcomes you have had to accept for yourself or your loved ones and how that might affect your thinking about your health today.

)(

Day 3
Tell Yourself the Truth

Facts do not cease to exist because they are ignored.

—Aldous Huxley

Being in denial about a situation makes it hard to take charge of changing it. It's a cliché because it's true: Accepting that you have a problem really is half the battle.

If you are in denial about either the seriousness of your condition or the power of your ability to impact it, you limit your ability to get healthy. Committing to taking care of your health will only help if you are honest with yourself about what actually needs to happen.

The tricky thing about denial is that, by definition, we don't realize we are in it. No matter how self-aware we are, we are almost always in a little bit of denial about any challenge. Not fully seeing how tough things are is a coping mechanism that can serve us well. When it prevents us from seeing reality clearly, however, it becomes a problem.

Martha E. Kilcoyne, author of *Defeat Chronic Fatigue Syndrome: You Don't Have to Live With It*, describes different types of denial when she identifies the following three responses to having chronic fatigue syndrome (CFS; also known as chronic fatigue immune dysfunction (CFID) and myalgic encephalomyelitis).[2] Although the issues differ for people with other long-term conditions like diabetes, heart disease, lupus, other autoimmune disorders, and some cancers, most of the same principles apply:

Response 1: What Illness?

"These people are often in denial about being sick or the need to follow any type of modified routine," Kilcoyne writes. They forge onward, seeing doctors, but aiming to alter their routines and habits as little as possible. Rather than looking for things they can change to take care of themselves, they often view any change or limitation as allowing the illness to win. This can result in years wasted trying to hold onto a reality that no longer exists, while doing ongoing damage to their bodies and missing opportunities to explore new healing paths.

It's understandable. When you have a new diagnosis or symptoms, it takes time to digest and accept your new reality before you can act on it. I spent a year or two in this stage myself. Don't be like me. Try not to be stuck here too long, saying things like:

> "It's not that bad."

> "I can still work full-time; I just have to rest all weekend to make up for it."

> "I've had to increase my medications a lot, but the side effects aren't too bad."

Response 2: Half-and-Half

"These patients get it, but only half the time," explains Kilcoyne. "They see-saw back and forth between adjusting their lifestyle to get well and jumping back on the merry-go-round...." This is a step in the right direction, but these folks still find it hard to accept the amount of effort or time it may take to achieve their health goals. I spent another two years in this stage as well. It can sound like this:

> "It's not that big a deal."

> "I've been feeling good this week. I can blow off my physical therapy."

> "Other people eat pizza. It won't kill me."

Response 3: Woe Is Me

"After struggling with CFS for a while, these patients accept their misfortune to have contracted CFS and seem to give in to a permanently 'sick' lifestyle," says Kilcoyne. They stop actively looking for a way to get healthier and mainly figure out how to adapt to their symptoms. This may sound like acceptance, but it can be a different form of denial—denial that there is more that can be done. It can sound like this:

> › "I've tried everything."
> › "I can't fight this battle anymore."
> › "I don't want to burden anyone."

After years of trying to get healthy, it is understandable that many people adopt some variation of this last attitude. They genuinely feel like they have tried everything and have no options left. But, don't let this be you. There is always something you haven't tried, support you haven't gotten, a different diet, or a new treatment to explore. Although it is hard to believe, just because the first 99 things didn't work, that doesn't mean that the 100th won't work either.

If this is you, try taking a break for a while from the job of "getting well," and look into getting more support to handle the tough emotions that make it hard to keep going. Check out Practice 2, Nurture Your Heart, for ideas on how to get that emotional support.

Lastly, the medical community even has a fancy name for helping people to accept their current reality and commit to changing it: Acceptance and Commitment Therapy (ACT). In short, ACT teaches patients to:

1. **Accept** their health condition and their feelings about it without judging them as good or bad.

2. **Commit** to goals for addressing their health condition.

3. **Take action** toward achieving those goals.

Research has shown that these three steps can make a world of difference. Diabetes patients who used ACT reported better self-care and lower blood-sugar levels months later.[3]

>>> *For Today* <<<
Explore where you might be in denial. Do any of the types of denial listed here resonate for you? What element of your reality can you work on accepting more fully? What support can you get?

><

Day 4
Jump In: Feel the Pain—Feel the Rewards

They always say time changes things, but you actually have to change them yourself.

—Andy Warhol

We would each like to think that we are the strong ones who decide to take charge and just do it, without all that messy denial. In reality, it often requires either considerable suffering, the threat of considerable suffering, or the promise of a great reward to motivate people to truly take charge and make a change.

This next exercise is adapted from Marilyn Paul's excellent book, *It's Hard to Make a Difference When You Can't Find Your Keys.*[4] In her book, the exercise encourages the reader to deeply feel how much they are losing by being disorganized and how much they could gain by creating more order in their life. Here you will explore how much you are losing due to your health condition and how much you could benefit by improving your health. It's not pleasant, but it's an important inventory to take. If possible, it's good to have some emotional support available to help you face these things.

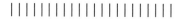

Step 1. Write down everything that your health challenge is costing you in each of the following categories. Write down every cost you can think of for each one. If your health challenge is not impacting you now, but will in the future if you don't address it, write down the likely future consequences.

Financial:

Family Relationships:

Friend Relationships:

Time:

Social and Recreational:

Work Life:

Spiritual Life:

Physical Well-Being:

Emotional Well-Being:

Step 2. Review each of those costs and, although it is uncomfortable, let yourself fully experience the loss of those things and the suffering it causes you. The more you let yourself feel this, the more motivated you will be to take charge.

Step 3. Now, imagine and write down everything that could improve in each of the following categories if you work hard and successfully achieve your health goals:

Financial:

Family Relationships:

Friend Relationships:

Time:

Social and Recreational:

Work Life:

Spiritual Life:

Physical Well-Being:

Emotional Well-Being:

Step 4. Finally, take a few minutes and let yourself imagine all of those improvements in your life in vivid detail. Let that motivate your healing work.

)(

Day 5
Jump In: What if You Accepted Your Reality?

Our lives only improve when we take chances—and the first and most difficult risk we can take is to be honest with ourselves.

—Walter Anderson

We often remain in denial to avoid what we might have to do if we acknowledged what was really going on. Use the following prompts to explore this. What would you do if you weren't in denial? Write down your first thoughts without editing.

If you answer many of the prompts with something like *I would curl up in the fetal position under my sheets and never want to come out*, it's a good indicator that you could use some more emotional support. We'll talk more about getting support in the next section, Nurture Your Heart. You don't need to do it alone.

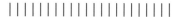

1. If I fully accept the seriousness of my health condition, I would:

2. If I fully accept how much time I need every week to really address my health challenge, I would:

3. If I fully accept how much money I feel that I need to fully address my health challenge, I would:

4. If I fully accept how much my health challenge is limiting my life and causing me to suffer, I would:

5. If I fully accept that achieving my health goals may require significant changes in my lifestyle, I would:

6. If I fully accept that the choices I make have a huge impact on my health, I would:

7. If I fully accepted how scared and stressed I am by my health condition and how those negative emotions might be affecting my health and relationships, I would:

8. If I fully accepted my power to improve my health, I would:

)(

Day 6
Become a Badass

They tried to bury us. They did not realize we were seeds.

—Mexican proverb

If you are having a hard time stepping out of some of your denial into acceptance, one reason may be because you are looking at acceptance as giving up—as passively submitting to an awful reality. That kind of acceptance might sound like "Wow. I am really sick and may never feel good again." No wonder you don't want to accept that. Who would?

That is not the acceptance that I'm talking about. That's resignation. I'm talking about an acceptance that is not giving up at all. It is about diving in. It's about loving and learning from all parts of ourselves. It is about becoming a badass. Like the seeds in the previous Mexican proverb, we human beings often grow the most and become the most powerful when we are buried in manure and have to stretch to get out.

Embracing your experience as an integral part of who you are right now, and learning and growing as much as possible along the way is a fast track to badass-ness. This doesn't mean you have to be thankful for your experience or that you should feel so accepting of it that you don't want to change it. It just means that you accept that this is part of your reality for right now and that all things come with both dark and light elements. Look for the light in this one.

You can use any religious, philosophical, emotional, or spiritual tools available to learn lessons and grow from your experience. In my mind, suffering through a major health challenge without milking it for all the personal growth it is worth is like paying college tuition and then skipping all the classes. You are suffering anyway, right? You might as well get as much as you can out of it.

In 2006, when I was at my sickest, I saw an acupuncturist for treatment twice per week. One day when I was particularly despairing of ever getting healthy, she said to me, "You will get healthy again and when you do, after all you've been through, you will be 10 feet tall and nobody will be able to mess with you."

I didn't believe her at the time. But I have come to see that the people whom I admire most and who move through the world with the most confidence and grace are often those who have come through some incredible trials, learned and grown from them, and come out 10 feet tall on the other side. In other words: real badasses. If you want to tap into your inner badass—if you want to be able to look any challenge in the eye in the future and know that you can take it on—do whatever you can to fully accept and learn from the experience you are going through right now.

Here are some examples of how others have received powerful life lessons and grown tremendously from their health challenges:

Rachel, 40 years old, living with Stage 4 cancer: "Let go of perfection." I do not need to be (and in fact, cannot be) the perfect mother, wife, daughter, and friend every moment of every day. The more I try to be perfect, the more stressed I am. The result is more illness and a crankier mother, wife, daughter, and friend. Faced with the ultimate consequence, I have finally begun to learn how to relax and accept that I am good enough, even if I do nothing for anybody and produce nothing. It has given me a deeper sense of acceptance of myself and others that can only be described as a gift.

Robert, 45 years old, living with lupus for 15 years: "Be the squeaky wheel." It is okay and sometimes necessary to make noise and annoy people. My illness was misdiagnosed for several years because my symptoms were unusual. I had to get over my fear of upsetting people and make some noise before I got the attention I needed, a correct diagnosis, and the proper treatment. I don't keep quiet so much anymore.

In my eyes, these people are badasses. They've faced some of the worst that life has to throw at them, embraced the challenge, and grown from the experience. I want to be like them.

You may also want to consider this: Many spiritual traditions hold that challenges come to teach us the lessons we need to learn and that we may continue encountering similar challenges until we learn those lessons. We could fill several books discussing the ins and outs of this position. Suffice to say that, if it resonates with you, you may want to internalize the lessons you think your health condition is teaching you, on the off-chance that it will help you avoid revisiting it all again someday.

Make a list of possible lessons that you could learn from your health condition and write down some thoughts of what it would take to help you internalize them and live them out.

)(

Day 7
Choose an Inspiring Destination

You must want it with an exuberance that erupts through the skin and joins the energy that created the world.

—Sheila Graham

If you haven't completely taken charge of your health yet, it may be because you haven't let yourself dream up an inspiring enough vision of what your life could be like if you did. We are much more likely to commit to and get what we want if we let ourselves "want it with an exuberance that erupts through the skin." That's a lot of wanting and a great deal more than we usually allow ourselves. It's scary to want something that much. What if you don't get it?

Most of us spend our lives avoiding humiliation and disappointment by lowering expectations and playing it safe. As a result, we don't get what we want or need, because we don't even let ourselves want it. So, just for today, try saying what you really, truly want for your health and well-being. Try creating what I call an Inspiring Destination.

When I was barely able to get out of bed for six years, my Inspiring Destination was: "I am healthy, energetic, and strong so that I can fulfill my potential and enjoy all God's gifts." That was my guiding light and motivation for all my healing work.

Stephen Covey, the author of *The 7 Habits of Highly Effective People*, taught that we need goals in our lives and plans of how to get there, just like a pilot needs a destination and a route for a safe flight. Without those, a pilot would travel aimlessly through the skies and wind up at a random location. Similarly, without a specific destination in mind and a plan of how to get there, we can wander aimlessly and never achieve our dreams.

Having a flight plan doesn't guarantee a smooth trip. Turbulence, air traffic, error, and other factors send planes off course frequently, requiring regular readjustments to arrive safely at the destination. Having an Inspiring Destination and plans to get there enables us to keep moving forward toward our goal, even when life's challenges throw us off course. An Inspiring Destination can help motivate and guide you every day if it is:

Ambitious: Make it something that you really want, even if you don't know if you can get there.

Positive: Rather than focusing on what you don't want, focus on what you do want.

Outcome-oriented: This destination is how you want to feel and what you want to do with your good health, not how many times you want to exercise each week to get there.

In the present: If you place your destination in the future, it may always stay there.

Inspiring: Use the words *so that* in the middle of describing your destination, followed by the things you want to do, feel, and be to remind you *why* it is important for you to arrive there.

Here are some examples of Inspiring Destinations:

› My sore knee is healed so that I can run and dance comfortably without pain or re-injury.

› I am at a healthy weight so that I can parent, work, and play exuberantly.

› Cancer is gone from my body, and I feel strong and energetic so that I can enjoy many more decades with my family and friends.

»» For Today ««

Begin to explore what you really want. Journal, talk with friends, meditate, or do whatever helps you think. Jot down some notes that will help you create an Inspiring Destination after you read tomorrow's story.

✕

Day 8
Melissa's Story: Shoot for the Stars!

There is nothing like a dream to create the future.

—Victor Hugo

Several years ago I met a woman at a health retreat whom I'll call Melissa. She had a shock of white hair and the energetic, muscular body of an athlete. I thought she was in her early 50s and was drawn in by her youthful energy and enthusiasm. I quickly learned that she was, in fact, considerably older and had not always had the youthful and athletic energy that I found so compelling in 2008.

Ten years earlier, she had been dozens of pounds overweight, pre-diabetic, and on medication for high blood pressure. At the time, her goal was to lose enough weight so that she could avoid developing type 2 diabetes, decrease some joint pain, and function better. However, she had a hard time keeping weight off and struggled to meet her goals.

One day Melissa went to a talk about healing and was moved by the speaker's exhortation to dream big. The speaker explored the idea that "people do not fail in life because they aim too high and miss; they fail in life because they aim too low and hit," a quote often attributed to the motivational speaker Les Brown. The talk that day explored how our attitudes and expectations shape our reality, and how what we expect with regard to our health is often what we get. He challenged the audience to dream big; to be brave enough to be honest about what they really wanted, rather than what they thought they could get; and then to go for that greater goal.

Melissa went home that night and changed her aim for her health. Rather than wanting to get just a bit healthier, she decided that she wanted to become an athlete—someone who was both physically strong and had great endurance. She had not been particularly athletic as a young person and her only exercise as an adult was walking her dog. But she decided that she wanted to be strong in a way that she never had been before. She felt like she was finally letting her real self shine through.

Melissa changed the course of her life forever. After months of research and medical consultations and more months of experimenting, she eventually settled on following a high-protein, anti-inflammatory, plant-based diet, combined with lots of yoga, walking, and swimming. By the time I met her, she had been practicing that lifestyle for years and her high blood pressure and blood sugar were things of the past. She showed me old pictures of her that were unrecognizable, more for the increased joy on her face than for the decreased weight on her body.

I learned from Melissa the power of choosing an inspiring destination and going for it, rather than just working to get by, and I am forever grateful for having met her.

»» For Today ««

Using the description from yesterday, create an Inspiring Destination and post it in your bathroom, bedroom, workspace, or kitchen to remind you of your heart's desire. If you doubt your ability to achieve it now, don't worry. You can also create smaller, shorter-term goals along the way.

)(

Day 9
Embrace Change

The only constant in life is change.

—Heraclitus of Ephesus

One thing that often prevents people from fully taking charge of their healing is a fear of change. Change can be scary. It involves risk and unknown outcomes. I can relate. It took me five years until I was ready to take on the diet that ultimately healed me. No judgment here.

What we need to face is that life is change. Right now as you read this, wherever you are on the health continuum, cells in your body are growing, dying, and reproducing in countless ways. In your home and workplace, relationships are always evolving as each person grows and your lives together transform. Around the world, new technologies, philosophies, and social movements are constantly being created. Rather than be afraid of making a change, it would make more sense to be afraid that we won't be able to change fast enough to keep up with all that is happening around us.

Take Charge

Experiencing a change in one's life, whether it seems to be for the bad or the good, as a time to explore change in oneself is simply the healthiest, most productive way to respond. As Albert Einstein famously said, "We cannot solve our problems with the same thinking we used when we created them." I would add that we cannot heal ourselves with the same information, habits, and beliefs that allowed us to be susceptible to our current health challenge in the first place.

Often, in order to achieve a major goal, people need to shed some part of their identity or beliefs to open up new horizons. In order to get healthy, I had to go from a disorganized, cynical night owl who ate whatever I wanted to a super-organized, optimistic, morning person who ate only raw vegetables for a long time. I realize that can sound terrible on paper. But I wouldn't trade the good health I won for the world. You may not need to go through such a dramatic overhaul, but there is probably some tinkering required.

Whether it's Oprah Winfrey or Nelson Mandela, the most successful people in the world—the ones we respect the most—usually got that way by proactively responding to changes in their lives and environments, rather than passively letting the change act on them.

As we all know, that doesn't stop people from letting a fear of change get in the way of their healing. Eileen, diagnosed with hepatitis, didn't want to give up alcohol in case it made networking for her job difficult. Sharon had always mocked alternative medicine and resisted trying new "fad" diets or eco-friendly products to address her skin rashes. Jonathan, who had chronic fatigue and fibromyalgia, was afraid of appearing weak and burdening his family if he stopped working for one year to focus on his healing. Does any of this sound familiar? What change have you thought of, but are afraid to take on?

»»» For Today «««

Think of a time when you successfully made a significant change in your life, like a move, a new job, a new relationship, or something else. Are there lessons you learned from that experience that could help you embrace change now?

><

Day 10
Jump In: What's Stopping You?

Your life does not get better by chance. It gets better by change.

—Jim Rohn

Take at least one minute to write whatever comes to mind about each of the following questions. Don't edit. You might be amazed at what you learn:

|||||||||||||||||||||||||

1. What proactive change that I am currently resisting could I make to improve my health?

2. Why am I resisting that change?

3. If I were a friend of mine, what advice would I give myself to overcome the concerns that are causing my resistance?

4. What am I afraid might happen if I make the change?

5. How realistic are those fears? How might I handle those things if they do come to pass?

6. What benefits am I getting from not making that change and from having this health condition?

7. Are those benefits worth the suffering caused by my health challenge? Am I willing to give them up?

8. What benefits might I gain if I make that change and successfully improve my health?

9. Are the benefits I would gain worth the risk of making the change?

10. What's *really* stopping me?

)(

Day 11
Be Action-Oriented

Knowing trees, I understand the meaning of patience.
Knowing grass, I can appreciate persistence.

—Hal Borland

Let's assume that you feel ready to make some significant changes and fully commit to your healing. Done, right? Nope. We all know it's not that simple. It can take a serious process to get there. Being compassionate with yourself, combined with having a bias toward action, can help you succeed.

The Stages of Change Model was developed to describe the process it takes to adopt a new behavior like quitting smoking, changing eating habits, and other lifestyle modifications. It shows how most people alter their behavior gradually, going through these five stages and often several periods of relapse before successfully making a new behavior stick:[5]

Pre-contemplation: Unaware of the need for change or unwilling to do it.

Contemplation: Considering the need for change and what it might be.

Preparation: Choosing a change and getting ready to adopt it.

Action: Taking the actions necessary to make the change.

Maintenance: Continuing actions and adjusting as necessary to sustain the change.

Relapse—or returning to old habits—is a natural and inevitable part of the process of change and can act on any of the five stages. Most smokers quit several times before they finally succeed, and it usually takes several tries to keep weight off after altering one's diet.

Relapse will probably affect you, too. I know I've had to cut sugar out of my diet more times than I can count. (How does it keep getting back in there?) The key to successfully making a change is not just staying on the wagon; it's figuring out why you fell off and then climbing back on—as many times as it takes.

Here is what the five stages of change could look like, relapse and all:

Pre-contemplation: When Angelina was first diagnosed with Parkinson's disease, she relied entirely on medications for symptom-management.

Contemplation: As her symptoms got more severe and she needed more medication over the next two years, Angelina began investigating other ways to manage her symptoms.

Preparation: Eventually, Angelina took her doctor's advice and got a referral for physical therapy at a full-service gym.

Action: Angelina worked with a physical therapist to establish a work-out routine that she could do three times per week, along with cycling or yoga three times per week.

Maintenance: Angelina put three gym workouts and three cycling or yoga sessions into her schedule every week, for a total of six weekly exercise sessions.

Relapse: Due to family or work obligations, Angelina often skipped her exercise sessions and had only two or three total sessions per week, which was not enough to improve her health the way she wanted.

Getting back on the wagon: This is the hardest part. After all that, who wants to start again? At this point, Angelina could either get frustrated and give up, or she could move exercise up in her priorities, get some support to figure out what was getting in the way, and try again.

The keys to making it through the Stages of Change are being compassionate with yourself when you are stuck, and then moving back into action. This does not mean letting yourself off the hook, but rather avoiding beating yourself up. Explore, without judgment, what went wrong and take action again as soon as possible.

After several more tries, Angelina realized that family and work would always win over exercise unless she made time for them. First, she asked her spouse for time in the morning to exercise. Then, she used a combination of workout buddies and prepaid classes to make her more accountable. She also had good conversations with her coworkers and friends to ask for their encouragement and logistical support in making sure she prioritized exercise.

It took longer than she had hoped to find a routine that worked, but thanks to relentless persistence, Angelina did and was rewarded with added strength and one more tool to help her manage her symptoms.

Choose a new behavior you would like to adopt. Where are you in the Stages of Change? Have you experienced some relapse? Take a compassionate look at the situation and ask yourself what is getting in the way of moving forward and what is one action that you can take to get back on track?

)(

Day 12
Commit

Without commitment, you cannot have depth in anything, whether it's a relationship, a business, or a hobby.

—Neil Strauss

The next step in taking charge of your health is making a fierce commitment to your healing work. That means prioritizing it, taking risks, and getting support to succeed.

For many people, making a commitment can sound scary or off-putting. *I don't want to commit. That's too big of a commitment for me. He's not ready for a commitment.* These are all common phrases that reinforce this sense of commitment as a frightening, weighty thing.

It's true that making a big commitment is difficult. It can require giving up things. It can cause conflict, shake your sense of self, and bring up tough emotions. But it's worth it because commitment is the secret sauce that makes everything better.

The more you commit, the greater the reward in any endeavor. Whether it's a relationship, a job, a spiritual path, or an athletic feat, committing deeply and giving it the attention it requires will make it go better and potentially bring you many levels of joy.

So, what does making a commitment look like? Like all growth, it happens in stages and it's different for everybody.

I knew that I had made a big step in accepting the seriousness of my illness and committing to getting well when I prioritized rest and self-care by quitting in the middle of a project and disappointing a lot of people. In the spring of 2006, I was leading my sons' preschool in a major fund-raising effort as a paid consultant, even though I was weak and achy all the time.

Two months into the nine-month project, I developed a low fever and body-wracking coughs that lasted for months. So I did something I had never done before: I quit. I could have kept leading the project. But I couldn't keep doing it, parent my children, and take care of my health at the same time. I cried buckets, apologized profusely, gave them all my notes, and left.

It was incredibly difficult to admit how sick I was and how much attention my healing required. But it was the beginning of acknowledging the seriousness of my situation and what it would take to get out of it.

Don't just take it from me. The medical community has also identified commitment as one of the keys to health. Since the 1970s, it has been recognized in decades of research as one of the "three Cs" of what is called *stress hardiness*, or how well a person can manage change and stay healthy in the process:[6]

Commitment: Enthusiasm to get involved fully with any effort they have undertaken and with the environment around them.

Control: A belief in one's ability to influence events in one's life.

Challenge: A proactive approach to change as an opportunity to learn and grow, rather than as a threat to one's safety.

Whatever you are creating in your life, commitment is an essential ingredient. To the extent that you already make things happen, achieve your goals, and nurture loving relationships, you have demonstrated the value of commitment. Now you can make sure that you are as committed as possible to achieving your health goals as well.

>>> *For Today* <<<
How do you feel about commitment in general? How do you feel about committing more deeply to your healing work? What emotions or logistics get in the way and what can you do about that?

><

Day 13
Jump In: How Committed Are You?
Commitment is an act, not a word.

—Jean-Paul Sartre

Take Charge

Commitment is demonstrated through action. Review the following list and put a check by the actions that you do now or have already done to some extent. Then go back and circle the ones you would *like* to do. Celebrate what you are doing and keep in mind where you'd like to grow.

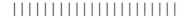

— I learn everything I can about my health challenge.

— I learn everything I can about conventional medical treatments and their effectiveness and side effects.

— I have clear communication and an excellent working relationship with my healthcare providers.

— I learn everything I can about alternative and supplementary treatments, and their effectiveness and side effects.

— I look into how diet could affect my health and make changes accordingly.

— I learn about how improved sleep could affect my health and work to improve the quality of my sleep.

— I look into how exercise could improve my health and work to implement that information.

— I look for people who have achieved optimal health with the same health challenge as me, in order to learn from them.

— I have emotional support systems to help me avoid being derailed by the tough emotions that come up.

— I have logistical support systems (child and eldercare, food preparation, shopping, etc.) to help me accomplish all that I need to do.

— I am open to the possibility of trying new things and making major changes in my life in order to improve my health.

><

Day 14
Set Limits to Set You Free

*Besides the noble art of getting things done, there is the
noble art of leaving things undone. The wisdom of life
consists in the elimination of nonessentials.*

—Lin Yutang

One reason that people are often afraid of committing themselves to a
new behavior is that it can require putting limits on themselves. If you get
married, you won't be dating that cutie in the next cubicle. If you take on a
big new job, you will be spending less time hanging out with friends while
you learn the ropes.

Getting married or taking a new job is pretty common, and so is the
support we get from the people around us to make those commitments
work. On the other hand, there is often less support to make more uncommon commitments with their accompanying limits, like choosing to avoid
wheat or sugar, making daily exercise a practice, or adopting a strict healing regimen.

Lifestyle limits also feel difficult for most of us because from the time
we were old enough to turn on the TV, we were taught that limits of any
kind make our life worse, not better. It is hard to make limits sexy in a
supersized, superhero, box-store world that tells us that we should be able
to have everything we want, when we want it. If everyone around us gets to
eat pizza and stay up late, we are afraid that we will miss out (or worse, not
be loved), if we choose not to anymore.

What the supersized world fails to teach us is the very basic fact that
putting limits on ourselves is necessary to create anything significant. The
limits themselves can often give us the focus to fly. Think of gold-medal
athletes. They missed out on a lot of teenage fun while they spent hours
perfecting their vaults, races, and flips. But they chose those limits to
achieve a greater goal and are usually thrilled with the results.

If you're inspired more by spirit than by sport, consider this: In the
Jewish mystical tradition of Kabbalah, accepting limits on oneself is not
only a positive thing, it is one of the most divine acts a human being can
do. Kabbalistic teachings say that before the world was created, God was
everything. There was nothing but divine power. Then God contracted

and made space for the creation of the universe. The Creator had to limit itself in order to produce the greatest creation. According to that way of thinking, limiting oneself isn't weak; it's the original act that led to the greatest expansiveness: the creation of the world.

Anyone who is in a healthy marriage or parents a child recognizes this phenomenon of putting limits in place in order to create something greater than ourselves. Giving up most of our free time and a big chunk of our sleep while we parent young children can be a huge drag, but the loving family we create is so worth it. So, I encourage you to see any limit required for your full healing as a sign of your power to ultimately expand, to take up new space, and to create the life that you really deserve.

>>> *For Today* <<<
Journal or talk with a friend about how you feel about setting limits and making commitments in your life. Does that attitude serve you? Is it getting you where you want to go?

×

Day 15
Make Your Choices Count

We don't have a live choice about every aspect of our lives, but there is always at least one point where we do have choice. We can identify that point and grow from there.

—Rabbi David Jaffe

Making a commitment can be hard. If you've ever made a New Year's resolution, you know that *sticking* to a commitment can be even harder. Today, I want to share a tool to help with that: the choice point.

Remember the scenes in old *Tom and Jerry* cartoons with the little devil and the little angel on Tom's shoulders arguing over whether he should squash Jerry with a frying pan? We all have some version of those voices arguing in our head all day. The Jewish system for ethical and spiritual growth, *Mussar,* calls those arguments "choice points" and encourages us to harness them as a powerful tool.[7] Here are some health-related examples:

Little Angel: The alarm clock went off. It's time to get
to the gym!

Little Devil: Relax. Skipping just one day won't hurt.

Little Angel: I'm having the fruit salad instead of
that cake.

Little Devil: It's a special occasion. Live a little!

You get the picture.

In these choice points, your healthier, more Divine-connected instincts that see the big picture and yearn for a life full of health, connection, and creativity are battling with your more base instincts of comfort, greed, and habit. You get to choose which instincts to follow.

Sometimes there is no choice point. Rabbi Eliyahu Dessler, a 20th-century scholar and leader in the *Mussar* movement, likened the development of character traits to a battlefield. If you haven't made a commitment to daily exercise yet, even though you know it would make a difference, then you are still behind the lines of the battle on the side of your more base instincts, where no fighting is taking place yet. There is no active choice being made. On the other hand, if you have spent months creating an exercise routine to care for your health that you wouldn't think of ditching, then you are behind the lines on the more Divinely connected side, have already gained that territory for yourself, and need not make an active choice anymore.

The choice points come at the front lines of the battle—when you have decided to take on your baser instincts and follow a healthier, more life-connected path, but haven't quite solidified that new habit or character trait yet. There is still a struggle each time you face a choice.

The beauty of this is, as Rabbi Dessler says, "If one side gains a victory at the front and pushes the enemy back, the position of the battlefront will have changed."[8] In other words, every time that you experience a certain choice point and choose the more life-affirming, healing option, you gain ground. Every time you choose patience over frustration, hope over despair, or a hearty salad over lasagna, it becomes easier to do it the next time, until it can become almost no battle at all.

Choose one area of your life—relationships, exercise, work habits, or eating—and notice where some key choice points are during your day. How much of a struggle is it to follow your healthier instincts? Rather than rushing through those moments, notice which path you choose. Noticing that you are making a choice is a first step to making healthier choices in the future.

)(

Day 16
Activate Your Body's Healing Powers

The individual who says it is not possible should move out of the way of those doing it.

Tricia Cunningham

The human body has an incredible capacity for healing when given the right raw materials. In our 21st-century world, however, we are faced with unprecedented levels of stress, environmental toxicity, and unhealthy eating and exercise habits that get in the way. The good news is that we can choose to stimulate that healing capacity through lifestyle changes that can propel us toward our optimal health in amazing ways.

Be Physically Active

According to the National Institutes of Health, "Exercise not only helps your immune system fight off simple bacterial and viral infections, it decreases your chances of developing heart disease, osteoporosis, and cancer." Exactly how exercise supports your immune system is not well understood, but it is thought that being physically active may help flush bacteria and carcinogens out of the body by increasing output of wastes like urine and sweat, and also helps circulate antibodies and white blood cells more effectively to combat bacterial and viral intruders.[9]

In addition, recent studies have found that the hours that most Americans spend sitting each day are taking their toll. Research shows that sitting for long periods of time contributes to cardiovascular disease, cancer, type 2 diabetes, and premature death in general.[10] The negative health effects of sitting all day are being compared to the dangers of smoking. [11] Even regular exercise provides only minimal protection from its damaging impact.[12]

Doing whatever you can to incorporate more movement and less sitting into your life can give a major boost to your body's healing power. Active hobbies, a standing desk, regular movement breaks, and walking instead of driving are just some ways to move more.

Reduce Your Exposure to Toxins

Time magazine reported that "A recent bio-monitoring survey by the Centers for Disease Control and Prevention (CDC) found traces of 212 environmental chemicals in Americans— including toxic metals like arsenic and cadmium, pesticides, flame retardants and even perchlorate, an ingredient in rocket fuel."[13] Arsenic can interfere with the glucocortoid system that helps regulate metabolism, which can in turn lead to immuno-suppression and insulin resistance. Flame retardants and perchlorate have been shown to disrupt the thyroid hormones that also impact metabolism and the immune system.[14] A trace of one of these toxins may be benign, but the current science is unable to tell us the health impact of exposure to low levels of multiple toxic substances.

If you're working to heal, you can choose to reduce the impact of this chemical cocktail. You can avoid many potential toxins by using natural household and personal-care products, using a water filter, eating organic, and avoiding processed foods. Eating the right foods and getting plenty of exercise and rest can help your body flush out the toxins you can't avoid.

Adopt a Healing Diet

Throughout history all cultures have turned to food for healing. Ginger calms the stomach. Garlic fights infection. Radishes help clean out the kidneys and liver. Unfortunately, today's basic Western diet is high in carbohydrates, meat, added sugar, dairy products, and refined grains, and has led to increased cancer, high blood pressure, obesity, and diabetes. The vegetables most commonly eaten in the United States are corn and potatoes. Even if you strive for a healthier diet, you may not be getting a big dose of vegetables like leafy greens, cabbages, or sprouts that contain antioxidants and other nutrients that strengthen the immune system.

Significantly improving your diet can completely change the building blocks your immune system is working with and increase its effectiveness enormously.

I could spend hours sharing stories of people who, in consultation with their doctors, addressed their health conditions primarily through lifestyle changes that optimized their immune systems:

> Debbie resolved years of undiagnosed, paralyzing back and joint pain by switching to natural versions of all her personal care and household products, increasing her vegetable intake, and cutting out processed food and added sugar.

> Allen got off his blood pressure and cholesterol medication by committing to daily vigorous exercise, reducing his daily calories, and increasing his daily vegetable intake.

> Sarah reduced her blood sugar and type 2 diabetes medication dosage by switching to a primarily plant-based, low-carb diet supplemented by high-protein vegetable juices.

> Belle ended all her debilitating arthritis pain when, at 60, she switched to an anti-inflammatory, primarily plant-based diet and began a regular yoga practice.

> Jamal significantly reduced his medication for multiple sclerosis and improved his mobility when he cut added sugar and processed food from his diet and worked intensively with his physical therapist.

I've experienced this as well. Annual bouts of strep throat or bronchitis and low-level fatigue bothered me my whole life. In addition to healing entirely from six years of illness, in the seven years since I reduced animal products, sugar, and wheat, and vastly increased the amount of fresh vegetables I eat and how much I exercise, I have not been sick with anything more than a couple of stomach bugs and a short cold or two. It feels like I was issued a new body.

I am not suggesting that you should forego conventional Western medicine. We are fortunate to live in a time when innovative medicines and medical procedures prolong life every day. Get good medical advice. But also do everything you can to support your body's natural healing processes. Many illnesses like digestive disorders, autoimmune diseases, diabetes, and high blood pressure can often be brought under control or significantly impacted through lifestyle changes. It is important to recognize that relying exclusively on medications, surgeries, or alternative treatments for healing can lead to putting off the personal changes that can bring you the deepest healing in the long run.

I want to acknowledge that it takes experimentation and a lot of support to sort through the overwhelming advice about diet, exercise, and healing. Start off with baby steps, get friends involved, and don't give up. I tried three other healing diets and concluded that nutrition had only a marginal effect on my health before I finally found the diet and lifestyle that enabled me to fully heal.

»» For Today ««

Explore new ideas about how nutrition and exercise affect your health. Do an Internet search of healing lifestyles like vegan diets, raw foods, the paleo diet, the body ecology diet, Ayurveda healing, and anti-candida diets, combined with your health condition, and see what you find.

)(

Day 17
Be the Boss of Your Healthcare Team

At the heart of advocating for yourself is believing that good fortune is always right around the corner, so long as you keep looking.

—Fiona Maazel in *O, The Oprah Magazine*

Physicians are usually talented, competent, and caring people who have trained for years to become experts in their field. We are extremely fortunate to have their skills and guidance. However, it would be a mistake to think of your doctor as the one in charge of your healthcare. That needs to be you.

Ultimately, physicians and other healthcare providers don't heal you. You heal yourself. The word *doctor* comes from the Latin *docore*, "to teach." A doctor is a teacher—someone from whom you can gain valuable information. Thank God for these teachers. Their knowledge and skills help save lives every day.

Consider this, however: Your doctor prescribes a treatment or performs a procedure, whereas you are the one who chooses the doctor and chooses to follow that treatment. It's your body that does the work to heal. It's you that has to make lifestyle changes and overcome emotional, physical, and logistical challenges in order to return to health.

Also keep in mind that every healthcare provider, whether she is a brain surgeon or an herbalist, is operating within a certain paradigm based on her worldview and how she was trained. Even when a provider does have knowledge about other medical specialties or alternative modalities, the 15- or 30-minute appointments she is allotted won't let her share very much of it with you. If you are not getting as healthy as you would like, you may need a broader perspective. In that case, throw open the door to a wider variety of treatment options than one or two providers can offer.

Being the boss of your healthcare team means handpicking your primary doctor after interviewing a few options, maintaining close contact with her and other providers to get their input, thoroughly researching conventional and alternative-treatment options, and getting your friends and family in on the effort.

You may already be doing a lot of that. Or, you might not have to do it all. But if your current efforts aren't getting the results that you want, you can step up your game by becoming the boss. Let's explore how.

»»» For Today «««

Get a jumpstart. Read an article or join an e-mail LISTSERV about your health condition. Start educating yourself more today.

X

Day 18
Ziesl's Story: It Was Up to Me

Life takes on meaning when you become motivated, set goals, and charge after them in an unstoppable manner.

—Les Brown

Sometimes dietary changes can bring miraculous healing. And sometimes you need to take charge and tell your doctor to find the horror-movie monster that is strangling your intestines.

Ziesl had had stomach pain for as long as she could remember. At four years old, she had surgery for a ruptured appendix. Throughout her whole childhood she spat certain foods into a napkin because it hurt too much to eat them and became a vegetarian at 10 years old because meat was too painful to digest.

Now Ziesl is a 40-year-old nurse practitioner and mother of two. Until recently, she has lived with persistent abdominal pain accompanied by acute, debilitating attacks of severe bloating and weeks of diarrhea. The acute attacks could include paralyzing pain, cold sweats, and fogged vision that immobilized her for hours:

Ziesl visited multiple GI (gastrointestinal) specialists searching for a cure. The diagnosis was always irritable bowel syndrome, which essentially meant "Your stomach hurts and we don't know why." The advice was to avoid dairy and be well-stocked with TUMS and Mylanta.

Over the years, Ziesl experimented with several diets. In 2009, a low-carbohydrate, whole-foods, anti-inflammatory diet made a real difference and reduced her symptoms significantly, but she was still left with persistent discomfort and some acute attacks.

With fewer symptoms on the new diet and more information from studying GI disorders, Ziesl developed a new theory about her pain. She realized that even when she went on a juice cleanse where she ate no solid foods for days and had no pain at all, an area on her right side was still always painful to the touch. She also noticed that her occasional acute pain was usually focused in that same area and would pass if she moved into different positions. All this led her to believe that she had an internal blockage. It was then that she went back to her physician and convinced him to do exploratory surgery. What they found was amazing. Says Ziesl:

> He found an adhesion, but not just any adhesion. Adhesions are usually thin, mucusy tissue from previous surgery that connects scar tissue to internal organs. This one was enormous. It had generated its own veins and arteries and tangled up around my right ovary, several loops of my large and small intestines, and part of my liver, and then pinned all of that

tightly against the right side of my abdominal wall. It looked like a separate organ—or something out of a horror movie. The doctors said they were surprised I could eat anything at all.[15]

The surgeon removed the adhesion, which seemed to have been growing since Ziesl's appendectomy 36 years before, and, just like that, the constant pain she had suffered for decades was gone. She has had no acute attacks since the surgery. The underlying food sensitivities are still there and she still needs to eat a very clean diet. But when she does, she says, "I am basically living totally pain-free for the first time in my life. It is just miraculous."

It turned out Ziesl's bowel was "irritable" for a reason. It took her doing her own research to figure it out. Her advice to anyone facing a difficult health condition: "Learn everything you can. Get all the help you can. Try everything and never give up."[16]

»» For Today ««
What could you do to learn more about your health condition or get more help to think creatively about how to address it? Schedule time in your calendar to take those steps.

)(

Day 19
Be Curious

To know what you know and what you do not know. That is true knowledge.

—Confucius

It may seem unnecessary in today's world to remind you to do research on your health condition. For many of us it is second nature to check in with Dr. Google as soon as we get a tickle in the back of our throat. But not all of us do and even those of us who do may give up too soon, not go far and wide enough in our research, or fail to follow up on all the ideas we discover. After all, it's not easy. If you do want to be the boss of your own healing, developing a deep curiosity about your health condition will take you a long way.

Here are some things you can do to develop your curiosity and satisfy it:

Make Time for Research

Set aside time each week to educate yourself about your health condition and all the ways available to address it. Explore the current research and new approaches to your health condition. Begin by typing a bunch of different keyword combinations into your search engine and seeing what comes up. Some useful keywords to search in combination with your health condition include *cure*, *clinical trials*, *studies*, *heal*, *treatment*, *manage*, *best tips*, *diet*, *exercise*, and *success story*. If reading is particularly difficult for you, ask friends, community social workers, or volunteers at a local organization for help.

Keep a list of treatments or approaches that you want to learn more about. When you come across something that seems too far outside your comfort zone, too expensive, or too difficult, don't disregard it. If it's really not something you want to explore further right then, add it to an ongoing list of possible approaches. That way, if you get to a point where you feel you need to try something new, you have a whole list of things to explore and discuss with your healthcare team that weren't right for you at one point, but might be now. Remember: The healing diet that helped me was on my "too crazy to consider" list for five years.

Question Your Assumptions

If you are a self-described "aspirin-phobe" who avoids the medical establishment and prefers herbs to doctor's prescriptions, open your mind to the possibility that there might be wisdom in the conventional medical world that you have overlooked. Remember Ziesl's story. After a dietary change helped considerably, it took surgery to resolve the rest of her digestive pain.

Similarly, if you are someone who only turns to conventional Western medicine, it may be time to broaden your horizons, step inside a health-food store, visit a yoga studio, or find a new alternative health blog. Dr. Mark Hyman's blog at *www.DrHyman.com* is a good place to start. He is a physician and one of the founders of Functional Medicine, which addresses the causes of disease by integrating conventional Western and alternative modes of healing.

It's also important to challenge your current assumptions about your health condition. If you've seen several specialists, tried a couple of healing diets, and seen two physical therapists already, you may think that no doctor, diet, or physical therapy could help you. That assumption could be wrong. You may just not have found the right one yet. Question your current convictions and keep searching until you find what works for you.

Find Your Tribe

It may not be appealing to you, but it is so important to take classes, join online forums, get into support groups, and generally connect with and learn from others who have a health challenge similar to yours. I know it's not easy. I resisted it for years. In the "go big or go home" world we live in, it can feel terrible to gather together with others who are facing the same tough times you are. On top of that, not everybody in support groups, classes, and online forums is upbeat, honest, and proactive in their healing. Sometimes it can be a real downer. Don't let that stop you. The wisdom that you can gain in some of those groups can literally save your life. Try to find one that works for you.

Jolene, a 65-year-old mom and retired bank manager, says that she might be completely debilitated by her multiple sclerosis if she hadn't spent hours on Twitter and online MS forums. She saw there that the people who were the most committed to exercise seemed to have the most positive outlook and often the most mobility and the best handle on their symptoms. It inspired her to work with a physical therapist to take on regular, vigorous exercise (weight lifting, swimming, and yoga) in a way that she never had before in her life. As a result, her doctors are impressed by how active she is and how well she is managing her symptoms. She credits her friends online with giving her the information and motivation she needed to get as healthy as possible.

>>> *For Today* <<<

Look at your schedule and choose a time this week to do research on your health condition. Explore ideas that you haven't been willing to look at before. Be curious about what's out there.

✕

Day 20
Make Good Hires

*If I had listened to the first doctor, I wouldn't be here
today.*

—Kris Carr

You probably wouldn't buy a new car without researching it first and
looking at a few options. But people do that with doctors all the time. A
2008 study of how people choose their doctors found that only just more
than a third used multiple sources of information to choose a new specialist. The study found that people were most likely to rely exclusively on a
referral by their primary care physician to find a specialist or to ask friends
for a new primary care doctor.[17]

In addition, once people choose a doctor, they are very unlikely to
change providers. This relatively passive behavior is completely understandable; medical information can feel so overwhelming. Starting with
a referral from a friend or your primary care physician is a great practice.
However, if you want to find the provider with the most skills, experience,
and success dealing with your health condition, some more legwork may
be necessary. Here are four things to consider as you look for the best doctor for you:

Track Record

Airlines publish their on-time data. Car dealers provide some safety
information. Yet, people often hesitate to ask doctors about their track
record. You (or your health insurance) are paying this person and you
are trusting them with your life. You deserve to know how they have per-
formed so far. How many patients with Lyme disease have they treated
and with what success rate? How many Parkinson's patients do they have,
generally how symptomatic are those patients, and why?

It can feel uncomfortable to ask these questions. Bringing a friend
or relative to appointments for moral support can make it easier. There
are also many Websites that provide patient reviews or background information regarding certification and malpractice history. Check out *www.
EverydayHealingForYou.com/Tools* for an updated list.

References

When companies hire new employees, they always ask for references who can vouch for the quality of their work. Why shouldn't we expect the same thing from our healthcare providers? It's a little out of the box, but it is so worth it. When I began asking healthcare providers to introduce me to people with similar symptoms to mine who had achieved total, sustainable good health under their care, I made better treatment decisions immediately.

Quality of Communication

Before anybody hires someone for their team at work, they make sure that they can communicate well with them. Do the same with your healthcare providers. "Studies conducted during the past three decades show that the clinician's ability to explain, listen, and empathize can have a profound effect on...health outcomes."[18]

How well you can communicate with your doctor impacts your health. Does she answer your questions completely, respect your opinions and concerns, and explain things fully? Does she welcome your full participation and exploration of new ideas?

Quality of communication also includes the ease of working with the office. Are you able to, within reason, ask a question outside of an appointment, deal with insurance issues, get copies of test results, and make and change appointments with relative ease? If the answer to any of these questions is *no*, if you don't feel completely comfortable sharing any concern or idea with your doctor and confident that you will get a thoughtful answer, it may be time to shop around.

Shared Healthcare Philosophy, With a Caveat

When hiring new employees, companies look for people who share the company's values and mission. Do the same. If your doctor turns quickly to antibiotics and surgery, whereas you prefer homeopathy and yoga, that's not a match. For your main provider, look for someone who shares your healthcare philosophy so that you are not at odds and constantly questioning her advice.

Here's the exception: When seeking a new diagnosis or treatment options, it can be extremely useful to look for doctors who use approaches different from yours or from each other's. Like Abraham Lincoln's "Team of Rivals," when you hear a variety of opposing views on a topic, it can help you open your mind to new ideas, clarify what rings truest for you, and collect backup options in case one method isn't working.

Cheryl, 40, used this technique to get advice on an old knee injury that made climbing stairs painful. By consulting with a chiropractor, an orthopedic surgeon, two physical therapists, a physiatrist, and a yoga teacher, she developed a well-rounded plan of treatment that included aggressive physical therapy, yoga, orthopedic shoe inserts, and surgery as a last resort. Happily, her knee was functioning well again after four months of physical therapy and she didn't need the surgery.

>>> *For Today* <<<
How does your current healthcare team stack up when evaluated based on these criteria? Is it the best team for you or is this a good time to explore some additions or other options?

)(

Day 21
Binyamin's Story: Don't Be Afraid to Fire Your Doctor

The minute you settle for less than you deserve, you get even less than you settled for.

—Maureen Dowd

Don't settle when it comes to your healthcare. Here is a quick illustration of how just one hour of research, some chutzpah, and the willingness to question a doctor made a huge difference in my son's life.

When my youngest son, Binyamin, was four years old, I suspected that he had a mild hearing loss. I took him to see an ear, nose, and throat (ENT) doctor who was recommended by our primary care doctor. The ENT specialist confirmed the mild hearing loss in one ear and said it was caused by chronic *otitis media,* or ongoing fluid buildup behind the eardrum. He recommended surgically inserting ear tubes to drain the fluid, resolve the hearing loss, and prevent certain, significant further damage.

After the appointment, I did some research, which means that I Googled *otitis media* and found that children with chronic *otitis media* usually have numerous ear infections. Binyamin, though, had only had one ear infection in his whole life. The diagnosis didn't make sense to me.

At our next meeting with the ENT specialist, when I began to explain my hesitation in accepting the diagnosis, he told me not to believe everything I read and emphasized again that failure to do the surgery would lead to further hearing loss. I was not convinced and went to get a second opinion.

The next highly recommended ENT specialist had a different diagnosis. He saw no indication of *otitis media* and said that the hearing difficulty was caused by a few bones in Binyamin's left inner ear that were even tinier than they should be. He said that the hearing loss should not get worse over time, that inserting ear tubes would accomplish nothing and that, short of getting hearing aids, there was nothing to be done except monitor Binyamin's hearing regularly. Later, when he is finished growing, he can choose to have surgery to address the congenital problem with his bones.

Now, seven years later, Binyamin's very mild hearing loss has stayed exactly as it was all those years ago. If I had gone along with the first doctor's diagnosis and recommendation, I would have subjected my son to one or two surgeries with general anesthesia and achieved nothing.

>>> For Today <<<

Is there anything about your diagnosis, prognosis, or current treatment plan that doesn't ring true to you or that seems like it is not working as it should be? Where could you look or whom could you ask to get more information or a second opinion on that issue?

)(

Day 22
Make Meetings Productive

The ideal doctor-patient relationship is like a meeting of two "experts."

Dr. Paul Haidet

I love today's quote. The doctor is an expert on the medical information she has studied. You are an expert on your own health, personal circumstances, and any additional information you have learned about your health condition. To get all you can out of your appointments, step into your expert status. Run your healthcare appointments like the health-care provider is a highly paid, expert consultant, and you are her client. You are paying her to advise you on how to care for yourself, but ultimately the final decision, the responsibility to follow through, and the task of living with the outcome falls on you. You are in charge. So, how do you run a productive meeting?

Set Expectations

When you make your appointment, be clear with the office staff about your purpose for the appointment and what information you want. Doctors make appointments of varied lengths, depending on the patient's needs. If you want a 45-minute conversation, as opposed to a 15-minute check-in, make sure that's what you are scheduled for. It is considerate of the physician's time and helps ensure you get your questions answered.

Bring Information

You will have more productive conversations when you have all of your medical information at your fingertips, and healthcare providers will take you more seriously when you are well-prepared. Here is a checklist of items that it's wise bring to every significant healthcare appointment in a notebook or file box:

> › Progress charts of your symptoms, if you keep them.

> › A copy of all relevant lab results and blood work for you to reference.

> › A copy of all relevant lab results and blood work ordered by other providers to give to the healthcare provider.

> › A well-organized list of questions for you to ask, with an extra copy for your buddy. (See the following.)

> › A short, written description of your medical history and current health condition.

> › A list of all your medications and supplements, with dosages and length of time you have been on them.

Bring a Buddy

I cannot overstate the value of having someone join you at any significant healthcare appointment. As Dr. Marie Savard (a national leader on patient advocacy) puts it, "There's nothing like having a friend or relative lending support, encouraging you to tell the whole story and helping you make sense of what the doctor says....I have found that the fear of medical findings can reduce even the most powerful, assertive person to saying, 'Yes, doctor,' and 'Thank you, doctor,' instead of asking important questions."[19] Your buddy can help you remember all your questions and make sense of the answers afterward.

Plan Your Questions

Set aside time before any significant healthcare appointment to clarify your goals for the appointment and develop a list of questions. It is important to know exactly what you want to learn in advance of the appointment. Some basic questions include: What are the risks of this treatment? What is your success rate? What does success look like? What are my other options, and what are their pros and cons? Why is this your diagnosis? Is there any way that my case does not fit this diagnosis? What are other possible explanations for my symptoms? Can I speak to others who have gone through this treatment about their experience? Remember: For big decisions, it's always a good idea to get more than one opinion.

Take Notes

One important role that an appointment buddy can play is note-taker. You can focus on listening and asking questions, and she can record the whole conversation for you. If you don't have an appointment buddy, make sure that you jot down key points as you listen. Statistics show that we forget as much as 80 percent of what we hear in conversations. If it's important, write it down.

Get Your Questions Answered

In today's healthcare system, most providers are overworked and have crammed schedules. Your time with them is limited. Make it count. Share your key questions with them immediately to make sure that they are addressed. If you sense that the appointment is ending without addressing your concerns, interrupt with, "Excuse me. I know time is running short and I want to make sure I get your opinion on this." If you want clarification on something, say something like, "I still don't understand. I want to make sure I get this right." If the appointment ends and you still have unanswered questions, ask how you might get those questions addressed.

Confirm Next Steps

Before the appointment ends, review and write down next steps for both you and the provider. That may sound like, "So, I am going to pick up my prescriptions and make appointments with the cardiologist, with the Heart Healthy program, and with you for three months from now. Your office is going to call me in a week with the test results and any other recommendations. Is there anything else?"

Do Follow-Up

Set aside time after a major appointment to organize your notes; write down follow-up questions; make copies and file new lab results; and schedule any follow-up tasks like researching a new diet, joining a program, or making appointments.

»»» *For Today* «««

What are some questions you would like to ask a healthcare provider at your next appointment? Start a list now so that when the time comes, you are already halfway there.

)(

Day 23
Manage Your Information

Information is a source of learning. But unless it is organized, processed, and available to the right people in a format for decision making, it is a burden, not a benefit.

—William Pollard

If you feel like you are drinking from a fire hose with all the health information coming at you, you are not alone. Between lab results, directions for medicines, supplement lists, physical-therapy instructions, surgery-prep instructions, diet recommendations, and your own research on treatments, the list is endless. Anyone would be forgiven for throwing up their hands and deciding to leave managing it to the professionals. But it's not in your interest to do that. They have dozens, hundreds, or thousands of patients about whom they are thinking and whose medication, symptoms, and lab results they are tracking. You have only one. They will do the best they can, but it will go better if you are tracking it all as well.

Having your information well-organized saves time for you and your doctor. If your doctor wants to see your lab results from a specialist, but can't access it immediately for some reason, you might not get her opinion for weeks. If you can hand the results over to her immediately, either as a hard copy or on a flash drive, *bam*—you're a hero and you get your answers right away. We've all shown up to a doctor's appointment expecting them to have received test results or other medical data from other providers, only to find that it never arrived. Don't let that be you again.

Healthcare providers can give you better, more accurate guidance if you make sure they have a complete picture. A 2012 study estimated that 5 percent of adult outpatients (or 12 million people) are misdiagnosed each year in the United States. One of the keys to addressing this is thought to be improved communication and information sharing between patient and physician.[20]

Here are three steps to tame the medical-information monster:

Step 1. Gather Information

Always get copies of every set of test results for yourself. You may need to push to get them, but it is *your* information. You deserve to have it. It is a big challenge for doctors' offices to share information effectively. Make sure that you have all your test results so that you can always give your provider what she needs. You can get them mailed or handed to you as hard copies, e-mailed in digital form, or handed to you on a disk or flash drive. If you have been at this for a few years, go back now to past providers and ask for copies of important results.

It is also very helpful to pull together the information that only you have, like your medical history and a current list of medications, and have it all in one place to hand over to providers when necessary.

Step 2. Understand the Information

Test results, medication directions, articles on new treatments, and other medical information can be confusing. Get help to understand them.

Ideally, have a copy of them in hand when you meet with your providers so that you can take notes directly on them. Don't be embarrassed to ask for clarifications or repeated explanations.

Step 3. Organize the Information

It is enormously helpful to have all of this information well-organized in one place. Although it may seem old-fashioned, a three-ring notebook or a file box can be the best thing for the job. That way you can look through items easily and quickly pull them out for providers to copy or review during an office visit. Having items on a flash drive for providers who store all their data online can be extremely helpful as well. In addition to the information listed in yesterday's entry to bring to all appointments, other items that are helpful to include in your notebook, file box, or flash drive are:

> › Your notes on each medical appointment, generally taken on the page of questions that you brought to the appointment.

> › Your research notes on various treatments.

> › Any articles on your health condition that you would like to discuss.

> › Tools like a pouch for holding business cards or brochures, pens for you and your buddy, and a three-hole punch for putting in new information.

If, like me, you are not a super-organized person by nature, ask a more organized friend or family member to come over for a couple of hours to help you begin to put your information together.

»» For Today ««

Get a notebook and a three-hole punch or a file box and folders, and begin putting your data into it in organized sections. Make one list of what information you need to get from where (like lab results) and another list of what information you need to create (like a list of current medications and supplements).

)(

Day 24
Put First Things First

Action expresses priorities.

—Mahatma Gandhi

We're approaching the end of Practice 1, Take Charge. We've covered several concrete things you can do to take leadership in your healing work. Now, how can you be sure to take action?

Once again, I want to draw from the wisdom of Stephen Covey in his landmark book, *The 7 Habits of Highly Effective People*. His third habit is "Put First Things First." By that, he means that once you know what your goal is, be sure to prioritize the actions that will get you there. Don't let other things get in the way.

What follows is an abridged and paraphrased version of one of my favorite stories from Covey's book about putting first things first. If you have done work on time management, you have probably heard this story before. Even so, it's always good to hear again. I know I need to relearn this lesson repeatedly.

A guest speaker at a university class pulled out a large jar and set it on a table in front of him in a lecture hall full of students in preparation to teach a session on time management. First, he put about a dozen large rocks into the jar until it was full to the top. Then he asked the students, "Is this jar full?" Predictably, they answered that it was.

"Really?" he asked. He then poured a bucket of gravel into the jar and let it filter down between the rocks until it was close to the top. He asked again, "Is the jar full?" Now the class had caught on and answered, "Probably not."

The speaker smiled and went on to add a sack of sand that filtered through the gravel and a pitcher of water that filled in all the air holes before declaring that the jar was finally full.

Then, he took a second, identical jar and added the sand, gravel, and water first. This time, when he tried to put in the big rocks, they wouldn't all fit.

He then shared with the class the point of the demonstration: "If you don't put the big rocks in first, you'll never get them in at all!"[21]

What are your big rocks? What are the highest priority items that you want to be sure to do each day, each week, and each month to make your life go well? If you don't schedule them in your calendar first and fit everything else around them, they might not fit in at all.

In order to overcome a serious health challenge, we need to make sure that the activities that promote our healing are some of our biggest rocks. We need to make them sacred items that go into the calendar, and let all the other gravel, sand, and water of our lives fill in around them.

Everyone has different big rocks, but some examples might be:

> Shopping for and preparing healthy meals.

> Making and attending medical appointments.

> Daily exercise.

> Taking supplements.

> Researching treatments.

> Researching healing dietary changes or exercise regimes.

> Joining a group or taking a class.

> Daily meditation, prayer, or writing.

> An early bedtime.

»»» *For Today* «««
Begin to think about what your big rocks might be.

)(

Day 25
Jump In: What Are Your Big Rocks?

The key is not to prioritize what's on your schedule, but to schedule your priorities.

—Stephen Covey

Take Charge

||||||||||||||||||||||||||

Step 1. Choose four "big rocks" that you could put in your schedule on a regular basis to support your healing. Look at yesterday's list of examples to give you some ideas.

Step 2. Choose the one big rock that will be the least difficult to fit into your schedule, and then note on your calendar when you can do it regularly, particularly this coming week. Maybe it's exercising three mornings per week. Maybe it's making a salad at home for lunch every day. Write it into your calendar as a fixed appointment. Let your family members and coworkers know, if necessary, to avoid being distracted.

Step 3. Tell someone who cares about your health that you are going to do this thing next week. Then, set a time to check in with him or her at the end of next week to report on how you did. Accountability is everything.

Step 4. Put another note in your calendar for two or three weeks from now, to add the next big rock into your calendar, and so on, until you've got all your big rocks in your schedule. Don't get discouraged if you put a big rock in your calendar and it "falls out" several times. It takes lots of trial and error to readjust your routines. There are some great suggestions of how to do that in Practice 5, Create Order.

><

Nurture Your Heart

*Every once in a while she'll get worked up and
cry like that. But that's ok. She's letting her
feelings out. The scary thing is not being able
to do that. Then your feelings build up and
harden and die inside. That's when you're in
big trouble.*

—Haruki Murakami

One of the greatest "a-ha" moments of my exploration into healing was when I realized that just because a person is afraid to take on a complicated new diet or unable to stick to a daily exercise regime, it doesn't mean that she is inherently disorganized or lacking in self-discipline. It means that something is getting in the way.

This is true for everybody. If there is something that you would like to be doing for your health that you are just not getting to—like making medical appointments, doing your physical therapy, or eating healthier meals—it does not mean that you are lazy or inherently disorganized. It means that some obstacle is blocking you from seeing and doing that which is one of the healthiest, most important, and divinely attuned things you could be doing: taking care of your well-being.

Sometimes the obstacle is an emotional one, like a negative body image that makes exercise challenging or a work ethic that makes any seemingly "nonproductive" activity like yoga appear worthless. Sometimes it's a logistical one, like not having time to make a healthy lunch. In this section, we're going to explore how to address the emotional obstacles to healing; how to nurture your heart and break through to the next level.

Day 26
How Emotions Matter

People who keep stiff upper lips find that it's damn hard to smile.

—Judith Guest

If you are having a hard time committing to your healing work, it means that emotional or logistical obstacles are getting in your way. The truth, though, is that it's mainly emotions. Most logistical obstacles could be overcome with the right attention and support—if our emotions didn't get in the way.

We might say, "The gym is too far," or "I don't have the time or money to make healthy food," but the reality is that if we had enough support and weren't afraid of change, doubtful of the outcome, or had some other hesitation, we could usually find a creative solution. The logistical obstacles are bigger and harder to overcome for some people than others, particularly those with few financial resources or significant physical disabilities, but anything can be possible if you get the right support and have the right mind-set.

I'm not saying that most of the time we have total control over the outcome of our health. That's way more mysterious. I am saying that most of the time, and maybe even all of the time, you *could* have more control over how you *take care* of your health, if some tough feelings didn't get in the way.

Keep in mind that those tough emotions are not your fault. You came by any emotional blocks you now have through genetic predisposition and events beyond your control when you were young. It can be hard to overcome them. However, you are the only one that can do it. And, once you do identify the emotions that are tripping you up and loosen their hold, the sky is the limit for what you can do with your health.

»» For Today ««

How does this idea that emotions are the main thing getting in the way of fully taking care of your health sit with you? Do you readily agree or feel some resistance? Are you excited to dive in and see what emotions may be blocking you? If not, why not?

)(

Day 27
When Feelings Rule Your Decisions

I thought by masking the depression with silence, the feelings might disappear.

—Sharon E. Rainey

We all like to think of ourselves as rational people who make decisions based on what is best for us in the long run. Sometimes we do that, but sometimes we don't. I often hit the *next episode* button on my favorite TV show, when heading to bed would be a better idea. I might eat a big dessert even though I won't feel great afterward. I don't think I am the only one who lets my emotions control a lot of my actions. Do any of these quotes sound familiar to you?

"I meant to go to the gym this morning, but I just didn't feel like it."

"I keep putting off that doctor's appointment. It stresses me out."

"Friends have recommended that diet to me, but it just feels too hard."

If these sound familiar, don't feel bad. We all let our feelings sabotage our best intentions. Sometimes we are aware of it and sometimes we aren't. A good rule of thumb is that you are acting based on feelings instead of rational thought almost every time that you reach for the less-healthy food, don't call the doctor when you think you should, or choose not to prioritize your health in any way. For most of us, that's a lot of the time.

That is not to say that we should never have a big dessert or skip a trip to the gym. It's just that when we do those things regularly or don't even try to make changes that could help us heal because they "feel" too hard, we are letting our emotions get in the way.

The truth is that even if you are well aware that your feelings are controlling your actions, it can feel hard to change. Finding a way to handle those emotions in a healthy manner can be tough. The first person who taught me about the power of emotions to derail healing efforts was my dad, Jim Hillis. He was diagnosed with pulmonary sarcoidosis when he was 69. That's an autoimmune disease that causes inflammation in the lungs and can cause difficulty breathing.

After his diagnosis, I did a bunch of research and found stories of people who had reduced their sarcoidosis symptoms through an anti-inflammatory diet that was high in vegetables and fiber and low in gluten, sugar, and processed food of any kind. I told Dad about this and encouraged him to consider it. But Dad had grown up in the 1940s in Nebraska and, in addition to being a class act and a brilliant man, he was a meat-and-potatoes guy with a sweet tooth. Although he and my mom did try to alter his diet a number of times, it was never a significant change; and it was no match for his illness.

His lung capacity continued to decrease and he was put on increasingly high doses of steroids, which had their own set of nasty side effects. The last time I talked with him about trying a more significant diet change, he said to me, "I appreciate your concern, and I know that changing my diet might improve my health. But every time I try to change the way I eat, I get depressed. So, what good is that? Would I be living longer or would I just *feel* like I was living longer?"

I tried to encourage him to find a way to deal with the feelings of depression instead of self-medicating with sugar and carbs, but it wasn't his style.

The last time I visited Dad before he died, we were sitting down to breakfast and he said to me, "I want you to know that I have taken to heart some of your advice. Now I have a bowl of high-fiber cereal instead of a cinnamon bun every morning."

He continued: "It works fine as long as I add a little of this on top," and he proceeded to squirt a spiral about 6 inches tall of whipped cream on top of his low-calorie, high-fiber cereal.

He always had an incredible sense of humor, which is one of the many things I missed about him after his disease continued to progress faster than the doctors expected and he died of lung failure nine months later at the age of 74.

>»» *For Today* «««

How easy or hard is it for you to think about changing how you eat to get healthier? If it's hard, what feels hard about it? What feelings does it bring up and how could you address those feelings?

)(

Day 28
Identify the Tough Emotions

We must be willing to encounter darkness and despair
when they come up and face them, over and over again if
need be, without running away or numbing ourselves in the
thousands of ways we conjure up to avoid the unavoidable.

—Jon Kabat-Zinn

It absolutely breaks my heart when I think about Dad's inability to change how he ate. I can't be sure that a significant diet change would have prolonged his life. I do know, however, that it was essentially not an option for him because he had no way to deal with the tough emotions brought up by changing his diet.

I don't blame my dad. I had the same problem. The healing diet that ultimately got me back to full health was recommended to me in the first year of my illness, but I barely gave it a second thought. Five years of illness and suffering later, I finally decided to take that original advice. Dad didn't have that much time. He died less than five years after his diagnosis.

Let's look at a case where identifying the tough emotions enabled one person to achieve a whole new level of wellness. Charles, a single, 40-year-old computer engineer, was diagnosed with rheumatoid arthritis. His physician recommended that he work with a physical therapist to develop an exercise routine to help manage his symptoms. His response was a fairly hopeless, "I'm not very coordinated. I'm just not into exercise. Maybe I'll try that later." Plus, the physical therapist that he was referred to worked at a gym and Charles hated being at the gym. "Working out at a gym is just not me," he would say.

Finally, a friend said something like this to him, "There is nothing about working out at a gym that is not 'you.' You just hate going there because you got bullied in gym class as a kid when you were a little chubby and clumsy. You're not that kid anymore. So, if you want to stay healthy and be able to work and live your life, you better get over it and get to that gym."

It took Charles a little while to integrate that powerful insight, but eventually he did and got himself to the gym. We don't all have friends who are that emotionally intelligent or in-your-face obnoxious. It's important that we do the work ourselves to explore why we aren't doing everything we can to take care of ourselves and then address that as best we can.

What outlets do you have for exploring the tough feelings that might be blocking you from moving forward in your healing? Do you use the outlets you have? Could you use more?

)(

Day 29
Use Your Neocortex

A man that flies from his fear may find that he has only taken a short cut to meet it.

—J.R.R. Tolkien

We often don't realize when our feelings are getting in the way of our healing because it's just part of how our mind works.

One theory of the brain's evolution holds that our brains are made up of three different parts that work together: the reptilian brain, composed of the brainstem and the cerebellum; the limbic, or mammalian, brain, composed of the hippocampus, the amygdala, and the hypothalamus; and the neocortex, the two large cerebral hemispheres. These parts of the brain evolved in order over time, yet are thought to still retain much of their original natures:

> The reptilian brain is in charge of the rigid fight-or-flight response triggered by fear.

> The mammalian brain makes snap judgments based on feelings and past experiences.

> The neocortex is capable of abstract thought, imagination, future planning, and advanced reasoning.

We hold in our mind all kinds of old fears and feelings that we've had since childhood, some of which we are only dimly aware. The problem is that the reptilian and mammalian parts of our brains respond strongly to those old feelings, as if they were current realities that need to be addressed.

We need to work on acknowledging those outdated feelings and fears, and avoid being triggered by them into either action or inaction. We want the brain of a highly evolved human governing our healing decisions, not the brain of a reptile that just crawled out of the primordial sludge.

How do you do that? You pay attention. Sometimes the ways in which our feelings can sabotage our healing are not concrete and are difficult to pinpoint. For example, I have a certain amount of free-floating anxiety all the time, which I trace back to a bunch of death and illness around me when I was young, combined with some other social factors. That anxiety leads me to feel almost constantly overwhelmed, even when there really is nothing to be overwhelmed by in the moment.

That feeling of overwhelm, in turn, often makes it hard to turn down a comforting bowl of mac and cheese to eat a salad instead. "It would feel so good to eat that mac and cheese...and I deserve it!" says the voice in my head. But that message is from my reptilian brain, or at best my mammalian brain, seeking escape from the old overwhelm and anxiety they sense. Those messages are in response to a 40-year-old feeling, not in response to the most finely crafted, creative plans that my neocortex can produce.

To override the reptilian and mammalian brains' automatic responses, you can consciously activate your neocortex to overcome those other messages. Recognizing that regularly choosing to eat a pile of starchy comfort food might not be a result of clear thinking is the first step in making the healthier choice. That recognition gives you a chance to move the front forward in the battle to change your habits.

»»» For Today «««

Think about one big or small change to improve your health that you find very difficult to make. When you think about doing it, or when you try it but fail, how do you feel? What are the thoughts in your head talking you out of it? What feelings come up for you?

)(

Day 30
Let it Out

To weep is to make less the depth of grief.

—William Shakespeare

Now that we've explored a bit of how your emotions might be affecting your healing work, how do you handle those feelings?

There are countless ways to address negative emotions. Different ways are right for different people. Here is a short list of some tools you can explore: meditation; prayer; talking with friends; individual talk therapy; group therapy; art, water, song, dance, or music therapy; alternative therapies like the emotional freedom technique (EFT or "tapping"), eye movement desensitization and reprocessing (EMDR), or neuro-linguistic programming (NLP); and journaling.

Check out any of these tools to find a means to identify and release the emotions that are holding you back.

>>> *For Today* <<<
Which of the previous tools have you tried? Which look interesting to you? What else could you be doing to ensure that your emotions support, not sabotage, your healing?

)(

Day 31
The Healing Benefits of Tears and Laughter

Crying wasn't like riding a bike. Give it up, and you quickly forget how it's done.

—Alice Hoffman

In my years of travel through the worlds of health and healing, one of the most powerful tools I have come across is the listening partnership. A listening partnership is an agreement between two people to take turns listening to one another as they explore their thoughts, feelings, and challenges. Although I have found many of the tools listed yesterday helpful, none of them has had the same impact on my life as this one. It also doesn't cost money and can lead to a deeply connected relationship that can enrich your life for years to come.

Deeply listening to one another has so much healing potential. It cuts isolation, enables us to work through difficulties, and connects us to our own humanity. In today's world there is little time to deeply listen to each other. Listening partnerships carve out the space to allow for that connection to happen. They also do something else that's pretty radical: They encourage people to show their feelings.

Our society tends to discourage big displays of emotion. If a person does begin to cry during a conversation, they usually rein it in pretty quickly. In a listening partnership, laughter, crying, and generally getting excited or emotional are encouraged. That's a great thing, because research has shown that releasing emotions through laughter and tears can aid in physical and emotional healing. It has been shown that laughter can:

> Reduce stress hormones and their negative effects.

> Stimulate circulation and aid in muscle relaxation.

> Increase endorphins, the body's natural pain killer and "feel-good" neuropeptides.[1]

Here are some fascinating findings about crying:[2]

> Biochemists have found that emotional tears excrete stress hormones that reflexive tears in response to an eye irritation do not.

> Typically, after crying, your breathing and heart rate decrease, and you enter into a calmer biological and emotional state.

> Most people report feeling "lighter" and more able to think clearly after having "a good cry."

So laughter and crying are both readily available, no-cost ways to improve our emotional and physical well-being with no side effects, but most people don't use them very much. Even people who say they cry a lot rarely get to have a really long sob unless there is some crisis. Why is that?

One reason is that people don't realize how healing it can be to release our emotions. We are all trained to think that crying or laughing too hard or too long—or sometimes at all—is a sign that something is wrong with us. That's a shame.

As very young children, we all easily laughed, cried, or yelled in response to emotional or physical challenges. If given loving attention, a small child will cry for some period after almost any emotional or physical injury, and then get up and be happily ready to move onto the next activity. Unfortunately, well-intentioned admonishments like "Don't cry," "Calm down," or "You're fine," teach us as children to halt our natural healing processes.

Those instructions to avoid showing big feelings come from the perception that the emoting is part of the injury and that, once a person stops crying, yelling, or talking excitedly, they are no longer suffering. In reality, the suffering, feelings, and beliefs caused by the injury don't go away. They are just stored away in our reptilian and mammalian brains and come back to subconsciously impact our thoughts and actions in the future. It is the crying, laughing, or excited speech that helps to heal the emotional injury and sort out our feelings about it. And it will help all the more, the longer it is allowed to continue.

We have all experienced a "good cry," where we feel more clearheaded and hopeful after airing hard feelings with a trusted friend. We also know that illness and its accompanying complications bring up a huge number of tough emotions. They can kick up feelings of disappointment, helplessness, and discouragement that often deeply affect decision-making, without our even realizing it. Listening partnerships give you a place to notice these emotions, work through them, and explore how they might be impacting your healing work in a supportive environment.

I am quite certain that I could not have changed my lifestyle and prioritized my healing the way I did without the support of regular sessions with my listening partners. Listening partnerships are a peer counseling tool used in a wide variety of health and educational settings. I will give an overview of the theory and practice in the next few days. If you would like more information, the most complete description I have seen of how to do them is available from Hand in Hand Parenting, a fabulous organization that supports parents to build deeper connections with their children. Their booklet, *Listening Partnerships for Parents: An Overview*, and self-guided video class, "Building a Listening Partnership," are great, thorough resources for anybody who wants to try using listening partnerships, whether you are a parent or not. You can order copies of both from the parenting tools page at *www.HandinHandParenting.org*.

»»» *For Today* «««

Think about how comfortable you are showing big emotions or talking at length about a challenge you are facing. How often do you feel safe enough to do either? When was the last time you cried hard with someone for as long as you needed?

⟩⟨

Day 32
Listening Partnerships: Not Your Average Conversation

We don't have to advise, or coach, or sound wise. We just have to be willing to sit there and listen. If we can do that, we create moments in which real healing is available.

—Margaret Wheatley

Although loving conversations with friends are wonderful and vital to your emotional and physical well-being, listening partnerships are different from everyday conversations in a number of ways.

Each Person Gets Equal Time

The two partners choose a place, time, and length that is mutually convenient for a listening session. They can do a mini session that is only three to five minutes each, or have a longer one where each person can talk for as long as 45 to 60 minutes. Sessions can be done by phone or video chat, although whenever possible, in-person is best. Using a timer helps ensure that each person sticks to his or her allotted time. By sharing time equally, listening partnerships help create a more equitable, balanced relationship and give each partner the safety to know that she has this time to use in whatever way is best for her. Occasionally, if one person is very sick or terribly upset by a recent crisis, it makes sense for their partner to give them "one-way time" and just listen without reciprocating. However, it's usually not a good idea to start off a listening partnership that way or to do that on an ongoing basis.

Emotional Release Is Encouraged

In casual conversation, we are usually hesitant to show big emotions and often quick to stop them when they do bubble up. In a listening partnership, showing emotion is great. You get to release old feelings that may be getting in the way of healing, with caring attention from your partner. In addition to laughing, crying, and talking, emotions can sometimes trigger long yawns or light shaking. These can both be helpful in letting the body release stored-up tension. As a listener, you can help your partner to let out emotion in a few ways:

> › Encourage her to slow down and not rush past descriptions of upsetting things by saying, "That sounds like a big deal. You can take your time."

> › Notice what part of a story triggers emotions, and encourage the speaker to return to it with statements like "It seems like there are a lot of feelings there. Can you go back to that?"

> › Rather than offer immediate comfort when tears well up, offer simple encouragement to continue with a murmured "Yeah" or "Go ahead."

The primary way a listening partnership facilitates emotional release is by maintaining what is called a "balance of attention." You've probably heard people in tough situations say, "Don't hug me or I'll cry" to a loved one. We've all experienced crises where we didn't really lose our cookies until we were safe in the arms of a trusted friend or family member. That's because in order to really let our emotions out, we need to both feel the hard feelings and feel safe enough to show them. By providing loving attention and confidence in the speaker, the listener provides the balance of attention necessary to allow emotions to risc to the surface.

»»» *For Today* «««

Imagine setting up a conversation with some of the elements previously described with a friend. What feelings come up for you? What would get in the way of you trying out this tool? How could you overcome that?

)(

Day 33
Let Structure Create Safety

Listening has the quality of the wizard's alchemy. It has the power to melt armor and to produce beauty in the midst of hatred.

—Brian Muldoon

When setting up a listening partnership session, using the following structure creates safety for each speaker and enables them to use the time effectively:

Recount a "New and Good"

After the two partners agree on how much time each person will take and who will go first, the first speaker begins her time by recounting something that has gone well recently. Examples could include a success at work, a heartfelt connection with a friend, or beautiful weather. This helps both partners start the session off on a positive note, feeling confident that there is good in the world and in the life of the speaker, before they dive into the harder material.

Review Current Challenges or Victories and Retell Stories

Next, the speaker begins to review any challenges she is facing or difficult emotions that she is feeling. She can either immediately go into detail regarding a specific concern or list a number of items and then decide which one to focus on. Examples of topics she could discuss include: fears about her health condition; confusion over which treatment to pursue; anger at her spouse for not supporting her healing efforts more; or anything else that is taking her mental energy. One doesn't always have to focus on current challenges. Sessions are also great places to retell and explore the impact of stories from one's life, and to celebrate victories as well.

Look for Patterns From the Speaker's Past

As the speaker talks about the current challenge, the speaker and listener both look for similarities between the current situation and any incident from the speaker's childhood or adolescence. A helpful question to ask the speaker might be "Is there any element of this situation that seems familiar to you from your past or childhood?" or "What was your experience with this when you were young?" This enables the speaker to notice where old experiences, feelings, and beliefs may be impacting her perspective on the present reality. It can be helpful to go back and describe those past situations in as little or much detail as is comfortable, and to let out any pent-up emotions that they bring up.

Return Attention to the Present

At the end of a session, help the speaker return her focus to the present, and reinforce the reality that she is safe in the here and now. As the listener, you can ask the speaker to describe something she is looking forward to, or ask a silly question requiring some creative thought to answer. A couple of examples of silly questions are: "Tell me three lies about a strawberry" and "What is your phone number backward and in Spanish?"

Using this framework to structure your sessions will help you and your partner achieve a high level of emotional safety and facilitate effective sharing.

»» *For Today* ««

Explore these questions: How might engaging in regular listening partnerships benefit you? If you aren't completely gung-ho about them, what is your resistance to doing them? Does that serve you? What other obstacles are in the way of doing them regularly, if you did decide that you want to? How can you address or get help with any obstacles to adopting this as a practice?

)(

Day 34
Practice Deep Listening

This is the problem with dealing with someone who is actually a good listener. They don't jump in on your sentences, saving you from actually finishing them, or talk over you, allowing what you do manage to get out to be lost or altered in transit. Instead, they wait, so you have to keep going.

—Sarah Dessen

Truly listening to another person is one of the most revolutionary things we can do. Thich Nhat Hanh, the Buddhist monk, author, and peace leader has said, "Deep listening is the kind of listening that can help relieve the suffering of the other person. You can call it compassionate listening. You listen with only one purpose; to help him or her to empty his heart…And one hour like that can bring transformation and healing."[3]

Let's explore how to evoke that healing through deep listening in a listening partnership.

Beam Caring, Acceptance, and Confidence

The most powerful element of a listening partnership is your caring or love for the other person. Through your body language, facial expressions, and language, let the speaker know how much you care about her and how confident you are in her ability to figure out her challenges and move forward in her life.

Be Quiet

Sometimes less is more. Often just listening silently to a person gives her the space she needs to explore an issue more thoroughly than she has ever been able to before.

Ask Open, Leading Questions

Only ask a question if it is to help the speaker delve deeper into her issue or clarify her thinking. Avoid questions that aim to either satisfy your curiosity or give advice.

Refrain From Sharing Your Own Stories and Experiences

Don't share notes from your similar experiences. It takes time and attention away from the speaker and is likely to take her focus off where she was headed.

Rein in Your Emotions

It's great to empathize when a speaker is sharing a story, but avoid giving big emotional reactions. That can shift the attention from the speaker to you and make it more difficult for the speaker to focus on her own feelings.

Avoid Judging or Giving Advice

One of the wonders of being listened to is that it can help us think more clearly and access our inner wisdom. Getting bombarded with opinions from the listener makes it more difficult to access that inner wisdom.

Maintain Strict Confidentiality

To create a truly safe atmosphere, commit to a double layer of confidentiality. First, this means that the listener will not speak about the content of the speaker's session to anyone else. Second, it means that the listener will not raise the topic of the session with the speaker in the future without asking permission first. The latter protects the speaker from being at an event with their listening partner and suddenly having an upsetting topic they worked on in their last session raised out of the blue.

It's not easy to delve into emotional issues, let yourself cry hard, or get angry in the best of circumstances. Add to that the busy, highly scheduled lives that most people live today, and it becomes even tougher to notice and release big emotions.

Setting up listening partnerships with people whom you know and trust can give you a much better shot at accessing and addressing your feelings so that your mind and body are as clear and fresh as possible to move you forward in your healing work.

»» *For Today* ««

Think about with whom in your life you might be able to share this method and try listening partnerships. List some names. Look at your calendar and decide when you might call at least one of them to share this idea. Keep in mind that when you start a listening partnership, you don't need to dive into the hardest material right away. You can begin with sharing stories about your life or your health and then let tougher emotions emerge naturally as you build more trust.

)(

Day 35
Rachel's Story: Thinking My Way Through Breast Cancer

The simplicity of it filled her with warmth. They had looked for her, and found her; she wasn't alone, after all.

—Laini Taylor

Committing to using listening partnerships on a regular basis to keep your mind as free as possible of old, damaging feelings and beliefs can make an enormous difference in how you approach a health challenge. Rachel found that engaging in listening partnership sessions regularly during her treatment for breast cancer enabled her to more fully take charge of her care, connect deeply to those around her, and recover more quickly in between treatments.

In December 2011, when she was 50 years old, Rachel went for an annual mammogram and found out that she had stage 2 breast cancer: a small tumor in her left breast and another one near her armpit. To treat the cancer, she had a total of two lumpectomies, five chemotherapy treatments, and 30 radiation treatments. She finished treatment at the end of August 2012, and will continue to take hormone therapy (pills) for several years to prevent a recurrence.

Rachel had already been using listening partnerships regularly for years to work through emotions and keep her mind as clear as possible day to day. As soon as she learned of her diagnosis, she made a decision to use regular listening partnership sessions with experienced listeners—people who had done hundreds or thousands of hours of listening partnership sessions in the past—to make sure that she could think as clearly and heal as thoroughly as possible throughout her whole experience. She spent several hours each week during her treatment in these sessions.

Rachel explains: "Most importantly, I needed to work on any old feelings and beliefs in my way of taking charge of my treatment, my health, and my well-being going forward. For example, before heading to the hospital for breast surgery, I worked on early memories related to hospitals, particularly feelings of terror and powerlessness. As a result, I was able to think better during my time at the hospital. I aimed to stay alert and in partnership with the doctors, nurses, and technicians."

Here are some other topics that Rachel worked on in her sessions:

› Deciding to put herself first, fight for herself, and fight against early discouragement and victimization.

› Her chain of memories related to cancer, including a friend dying of leukemia when she was a teenager.

› The physical symptoms and the feelings they brought up.

› Noticing that she was not alone and that she was cherished.

› Celebrating her victories.

› Facing her deepest fears, including what felt "unbearable," like death.

All that emotional work gave Rachel more flexible thinking and resilience throughout her treatment. "I was able to identify the old feelings and beliefs that had left me vulnerable to making mistakes in taking charge of my care," she explains. "For example, I noticed that I didn't like to call the doctor for extra help when I didn't have an appointment, especially on weekends or holidays.…[Because of old messages] I felt like I was being a 'burden' or a 'hypochondriac' or a 'complainer' or 'hysterical.' Over time, my judgment improved about which symptoms required immediate medical attention."

Rachel also used her sessions to help her manage her pain with few painkillers, and was able to keep her mind very clear and recover quickly throughout the treatment as a result. Says Rachel:

> It is impossible for me to know what my experience would have been if I had routinely taken painkillers or hadn't had sessions for hours each week. What I do know is that medical professionals frequently commented on how well and quickly I recovered from surgery, chemotherapy, and radiation. For example, I continued to work throughout my treatment—not every day, but on many days. Other patients undergoing similar or identical treatment were unable to do so.

> To resist victimization, and for the sake of my long-term survival and flourishing, I decided shortly after my diagnosis that I would not only survive breast cancer but would end the experience in better emotional and physical shape than when I started. I believe I have already achieved that goal in terms of liberating myself from a lot of old feelings and patterns of behavior. Physically, I am still recovering from the long-term effects of the treatment and hormone therapy, but I am hopeful that I will succeed in that arena as well. I am already exercising more than I was prior to my diagnosis, and I am confident that trend will continue. Of course, I will never be glad that I got breast cancer, but all things taken into account, I believe I moved forward as a result of the experience.[4]

»»» For Today «««

How does Rachel's story resonate with you? Can you imagine using listening partnerships to help you navigate your healing process?

><

Day 36
Reach for the Joy

My old definition of joy always seemed like it was in the future. When I get this, I'll be joyful. When I get that, I'll be joyful. When I feel better; am better; I'll be joyful. And it's sad to look back on so many days that I wasted waiting for joy rather than waking up to the fact that it's all around me.

—Kris Carr

Another powerful antidote to the fear and anxiety sometimes stirred up by a health condition is joy. And sometimes joy can feel in short supply when dealing with health challenges. If we want joy, we have to actively reach for it. We'll explore some ways to do that in the next few days.

Practicing gratitude is one of the most powerful ways to embrace joy. As Oprah Winfrey says, "If you focus on what you have, you will begin to see that you have more. And if you focus on what you don't have, you will always live in a space of lack."[5] Studies have also shown that consciously expressing gratitude can improve your physical health, quality of sleep, and self-esteem.[6]

One of the best ways to actively appreciate what you have is to keep a gratitude journal, in which you write five specific things for which you are grateful every day and spend a few minutes focusing on each one. It can relax you and help you notice the good around you.

Another way to appreciate the good in your life is a brilliant practice that Martha Beck calls "feasting." In her book, *The Joy Diet: 10 Daily Practices for a Happier Life*, Beck describes *feasting* as enhancing positive life experiences. She expands this description on her Website, saying, "The most common definition of the word feast, of course, is a large meal. Most Joy Diet feasts, however, don't involve food....Hearing a symphony or touching the curve of your lover's elbow could definitely count as a feast, provided that you pay the right kind of attention."

Beck explains that, to create a feast, "it helps to perform some kind of ritual that will direct your attention to the symbolic significance of your actions. A ritual, however simple, creates a border around an activity the way a frame does around a picture. It sets this activity apart from regular life in a way that emphasizes beauty and uniqueness, ensuring that those who participate in it become more aware of its meaning."[7]

In our home, having candles and flowers at the table can transform a ho-hum family dinner conversation into that kind of joy-inducing, connected feast. Similarly, playing music, singing softly, and waking up my sons with short massages instead of just yelling "It's time to get up!" can turn a key part of our morning routine into a feast instead of a fiasco. Look for spots in your life that can be enhanced to create these joyful feasts.

If you are finding it difficult to find any spots of joy for gratitude or feasting, you may be depressed. If so, you're not alone. Dealing with a long-term health issue can be depressing. I know. I've been there. When you feel depressed, dark messages and fears cloud your thinking so that you feel hopeless, discouraged, and unable to see much good now or in the future.

The Patient Health Questionnaire is a great self-assessment tool that, though not providing a precise medical diagnosis, can help you determine if you might be depressed. You can find the questionnaire at *www. EverydayHealingforYou.com/tools*. (Adjust the scoring accordingly if your health condition shares some symptoms with depression, like fatigue or difficulty concentrating.) If you think you are depressed, talk to your friends and family, get support, use the tools in this book, or consider seeing a therapist for help.

>>> *For Today* <<<

Choose an activity in your life that could be enhanced to experience more meaning and joy. Decide how you want to add ritual or attention to turn it into a feast.

><

Day 37
Increase Your Joy

You have turned for me my mourning into dancing: you have put off my sackcloth, and girded me with gladness.

—Psalm 30

Yesterday we talked about how to notice the joy that you already have in your life. Here are two suggestions for how to bring more joy into your life.

Laugh

We've already talked about how laughter is great for your health. The catch is that, according to some studies, small children laugh 300 to 400 times per day, whereas adults only work up a chuckle about 15 times per day.[8] The truth is that if you're dealing with a major health challenge, you may find that your daily laugh count is even lower. It's not always easy to find the funny.

In *The Joy Diet,* Martha Beck recommends getting at least 30 laughs a day and shooting for 100. I took her advice when I was depressed during my illness by putting together a "laughter kit" that included *Far Side* and *Dilbert* comic books, and DVDs of *The Simpsons* and *Seinfeld*. It sounds silly, but spending hours laughing with my kit, especially with other people, was one important piece to pulling me out of my depression. Try it. It can't hurt.

Do What You Love

You only live once. Making time to embrace the things you love can significantly increase your joy and reduce stress. Make room in your life for the things that you love and can do: art, music, carpentry, quilting, reading, dancing, writing, gardening, hiking, or whatever—even if it is only a little bit every now and then.

I want to acknowledge two things about this. First, though it can be fabulous for your well-being to do what you love, be careful not to pour your attention into a hobby to avoid dealing with the reality of your health condition.

Second, if you are dealing with major health challenges, some more physically demanding things like gardening or dancing may seem impossible. It can be difficult to accept limitations, but sometimes adapting your passions to your current abilities can still bring joy. If gardening or dancing feel out of reach, maybe having an herb garden in pots or dancing while sitting down would be good options. See what works for you and get emotional support to help deal with any grief you need to work through to get back to your passions in a new, adapted way. Plus, there are less-demanding joy-inducing activities to choose from like reading; singing; crafting; listening to music, podcasts; or audiobooks; and watching good-quality entertainment.

To see one of the most potent illustrations of doing what you love and reaching for joy in the face of a health challenge, look up the beautiful viral video "Deb's OR Flash Mob" on YouTube. When Dr. Deborah Cohan was diagnosed with stage 2 breast cancer and needed a double mastectomy in November 2013, she decided that she wanted to go into the surgery as strong, centered, and joyful as possible, so she danced—in the operating room, to Beyoncé, with a team of surgical residents and nurses grooving along with her. It is breathtaking to watch. As Dr. Cohan explains:

> I asked the anesthesiologist if I could dance before the surgery. I knew it was a crazy request, but I wanted to be in a really vibrant place and have my body be receptive to surgery…. Most patients get medicated and go in on a gurney. I wanted to have my fully conscious self walking in there, choosing to have the surgery…. For me, this wasn't about ignoring fear—it was about confronting fear and sorrow really directly. I was afraid of death, and once I really fully explored that—what it would look like for me to die right now and leave my two young kids—I just went there. And once I did, it was a discovery that while I had to have this experience, I was not going to die from having my breasts taken off. And then there was space for joy.[9]

»» *For Today* ««

Check out "Deb's OR Flash Mob" on YouTube and learn more about Dr. Cohan's perspectives on healing through joy and movement at *www.embodiedmedicine.com* and "Deborah Cohan's Healing Journey" on Facebook.

)(

Day 38
Find Joy Through Connection

But that's just it; I can either focus on what I have lost, or what I have gained, and I choose the latter.

—Angie Smith

When speaking about the feasting that we discussed yesterday, Martha Beck says, "In the end, there is one sort of feast that eclipses all the other kinds put together, and that is a feast of love… To me a feast of love is any instant (or hour or lifetime) when human beings exchange affection."[10]

One of the pitfalls of having a serious health condition is that you may miss out on a lot of love feasts. That can be very isolating, which can lead to depression and make it harder to take care of yourself.

Do whatever you can to connect with others and avoid that isolation. If you don't have the energy to go out, let your friends know how they can come and be social with you in a way that is not draining. Maybe someone could come watch a movie with you, bring a meal and eat with you, or bring a book and just read quietly with you in the same room.

Gretchen Rubin, author of *The Happiness Project*, says that the happy-making tip that she found most effective was to join or start a group. "We know from the research that what makes us happiest is strong relations with other people, and you can build that through joining or starting up groups."[11]

If you are well enough, getting involved in groups related to your health condition that have a proactive, positive perspective can be very rewarding. Catherine, 40 years old, had type 1 diabetes for more than 15 years when she signed up for her first Tour de Cure biking fund-raiser for the American Diabetes Association. One of their catch phrases is *Paint the Town Red! Do you have diabetes? Then you are a red rider. Be bold! Be celebrated!*

Catherine was surprised by how powerful it was to get involved with the ride. She explains: "It was revolutionary. To be celebrated for living with diabetes? I've always had so much shame around it and it has been so wrapped up in my own challenges with body image and people's misperceptions that diabetes is caused by being overweight. To be told to be bold about it and that I would be celebrated? It felt so good to be seen and to be recognized for the hard things I live with every day. It's a completely new feeling to be part of something like this. It's very exciting."[12]

If you are not physically well enough to go out to group meetings, look into joining online groups that relate either to your health condition, or to something else that gives you joy. Carmel, a physician in North Carolina, has two fabulous daughters, one of whom is severely disabled with cerebral palsy. Carmel says that her "online family" of other parents raising disabled children is her lifeline and greatest source of support. When nobody else understands what she is going through, she knows they'll be there. Look around to see what you like. If you try one and hate it, don't give up. There are a gazillion groups out there. There's one for you.

>»» *For Today* «««

Think of a couple of ways that you can connect with others in the next week, even if they are just small, first steps. Write them down in your calendar to help you remember.

><

Day 39
Create a Life You Want to Show Up For

To be nobody but yourself in a world which is doing its best day and night to make you like everybody else means to fight the hardest battle which any human being can fight....

—E.E. Cummings

In the first year of my illness, one of my all-time favorite healers, Dr. Heidi Fleiss-Lawrence of the Jerusalem Family Wellness Center, asked me something along the lines of "Are you expressing your will in your life and your relationships?" A couple of years later, a particularly insightful and opinionated homeopath put it more bluntly: "Are you living a life that you want to show up for?"

Deeply connected caregivers know that your emotional well-being is key to your physical well-being—that when significant elements of your life are preventing you from experiencing joy or being your authentic self, your health suffers. In Dr. Lissa Rankin's book, *Mind Over Medicine*, she talks about noticing a correlation in many of her patients between being meaningfully happy and being healthy. At first, when she began asking her patients the question, "What does your body need in order to heal?" the responses shocked her. Whereas some people responded with medical answers like needing the right antibiotic or wanting to get their hormones in balance, many more replied with answers like "I have to quit my job"; "It's time to finally come out of the closet to my parents"; "I must divorce my spouse"; "I have to finish my novel"; and "I need to forgive myself."[13]

Dr. Rankin tells the story of Marla, who was in an abusive marriage, had an unpleasant job, and had numerous chronic autoimmune conditions. Marla answered the question with "I need to move to Santa Fe." When Dr. Rankin asked her why, Marla said, "I have a vacation home in Santa Fe, and whenever I go there, all of my symptoms disappear." Sure enough, a year later, Dr. Rankin heard from Marla. She had moved to Santa Fe, divorced her husband, and started a new career and a new life. Her symptoms were gone. She was healthy and happy.[14]

Maybe there was a physical explanation for Marla's healing. Maybe there was an allergen in her previous home that was absent in Santa Fe. Who knows? But the thing is, it wasn't just Marla. Dr. Rankin "witnessed similar transformations in dozens of patients" who switched jobs, ended unhealthy relationships, or made other significant changes and achieved vastly improved health as a result.[15]

By taking some major steps, these individuals reduced stress, gave themselves more of those health-inducing hormones that joy brings, created lives they really wanted to be living, and freed their bodies up to heal in the process.

>»> *For Today* «<«

Ask yourself the question "What do I need in order to heal?"
Give yourself a chunk of time to think or journal about it.
You might be surprised at the answers.

)(

Day 40
Liza's Story: Choosing Joy

Joy does not simply happen to us. We have to choose joy and keep choosing it every day.

—Henri J.M. Nouwen

Knowing when to expend energy to reach for joy and when to cut back and conserve your resources is a tough calculation. During my illness, people often encouraged me to "go out and have fun" from a misguided perspective that I was tired because I was depressed and needed to be cheered up. Occasionally those outings gave me a renewed determination to get healthy, but more often they just sapped my already-low resources.

Sometimes, however, making a bold grab for life is exactly what is called for. The future remains unclear for Liza Heaton, but read on to see how she took her chance to reach for joy and what happened afterward.

On Saturday, December 13, 2014, Liza Heaton, 25, had just received devastating news. Less than a week before, she was told that a rare cancer called synovial sarcoma had returned after three years of remission, and she had only weeks to live. A chemotherapy treatment could have helped, but a gastrointestinal obstruction made the treatment impossible. Liza's oncologists in Baltimore recommended hospice and palliative care.

Liza gathered 150 friends and family in her home state of Louisiana to say goodbye, and surprised them with a wedding instead.

Liza and her longtime boyfriend, Wyatt, had spoken about getting married before. But "when they said it would not be months, but weeks, I took that to mean a wedding was off the table," Liza said. "Wyatt took it to mean, okay, we have to get married this weekend."[16]

The two decided to do it and, with just a few days' notice, were married at Cross Lake near Shreveport, Louisiana. The wedding was a spirited celebration, despite the circumstances. Although she had been bedridden most of the previous week, Liza danced and partied for hours, soaking up the joy and love she shared with her family and friends.

The day after the wedding, there was an amazing development in Liza's health. The obstruction that prevented Liza's treatment cleared and her oncologists were able to prescribe a chemotherapy pill that could halt the progress of the tumors.

Her family said that they hoped the pill would stop the growth of the tumors enough to enable Liza to join a clinical trial that could treat the cancer in the spring.

What was Liza's perspective? "Maybe it will turn around, and if it doesn't, enjoy what you have. Enjoy the time you have left," she said.[17]

You can go to *www.gofundme.com/loveforliza* (as of February 2015) to learn more and donate to the Love for Liza Fund at the Johns Hopkins Sidney Kimmel Comprehensive Cancer Center. The funds will be used for research regarding synovial sarcoma and all sarcomas in general.

Nurture Your Heart

We don't all have a fiancé waiting to throw us a wedding, but we do all have things that would bring us joy that we have put off for one reason or another. What could you do to remind your body and mind how connected you are and how much joy there is to be had in the here and now?

)(

Believe

*Every time you state what you want or believe,
you're the first to hear it. It's a message to both
you and others about what you think is possible.
Don't put a ceiling on yourself.*

—Oprah Winfrey

Now that we've looked at what it means to take charge of your health and some ways to manage some of the tough emotions that come up, this month we will explore how developing fierce confidence in your ability to get healthy can improve your physical and emotional well-being and enable you to pursue your goals wholeheartedly.

This is not just about having a positive attitude. In fact, if anybody tells you to "keep your chin up," you'd be well within your rights to punch them in theirs. This is not about living under the pretense that everything is okay. It is about making space for the tough feelings that come up, while simultaneously reaching for the joy, confidence, and trust that will keep you moving forward.

There is no correct way to do this. For some people, believing they will beat cancer looks like naming their tumor, thanking it for coming to teach them a lesson, then graciously inviting it to leave. For others, it looks like envisioning their cancer cells as enemy invaders and chemotherapy as a weapon of mass destruction. Some do a little bit of both. Often, accepting that you may not achieve your current health goal can be an integral part of committing to meet it, though sometimes it can take the wind out of your sails.

There is no right way or wrong way to believe. There is only your way: the way that feels authentically you, rooted in your best self, and grounded in love. This month we'll look at several ways to strengthen your belief in your ability to achieve your health goals. I invite you to explore them with this question in mind: "How will I believe?"

Day 41
Cultivate Your Inner Quarterback

*Life is not easy for any of us. But what of that? We must
have perseverance and above all confidence in ourselves.
We must believe that we are gifted for something and that
this thing must be attained.*

—Marie Curie

Believing propels healing forward like nothing else. I chose the word *believe* to be clear that I am not talking about hope. The attitude we are going for is not "I am hopeful that I will be healthy someday." We are going for "I am certain that I am moving unstoppably toward optimal health." We'll explore some of the nuances around holding strong beliefs and accepting limitations at the same time. For now, let's build up that belief muscle. If you are not there already, it will take some time and effort to cultivate, but every move in that direction improves your ability to reach your health goals, whatever they may be.

Many studies have shown that having a positive outlook can significantly improve health, from increasing immune responses and pain tolerance to preventing heart disease.[1]

This works on several levels:

> A positive outlook decreases stress and its negative effects on your body.

> You are more likely to work hard on healing if you believe you can heal.

> Your body and mind are closely connected. Your moods and expectations can impact your health in ways we are just beginning to understand.

This, then, is a good time to connect to your inner NFL quarterback. When he bursts onto the field at the beginning of the second half, he doesn't say, "I really hope we win this one" or "I think we can probably win this one." He growls, "Let's go kick some a**!" That's the tone we are going for: fiercely confident, not cautiously hopeful. That's real belief. And you can do it.

>>> *For Today* <<<

How strong is your conviction that you can achieve your health goals? What old stories or beliefs do you hold that might get in the way of fully believing? Are they serving you?

><

Day 42
Understand the Placebo Effect

We all know people in clinical trials get better when you treat them with nothing but a sugar pill. But why?

—Dr. Lissa Rankin

When you fully believe in your ability to heal, you give yourself a huge advantage. As long as you actively doubt that you can achieve your health goals, you can undermine your healing efforts. That the quarter-back "knows" he is going to win is half the battle. He wouldn't complete many passes if he was thinking, "I don't know if I can do this" as he tossed the ball. Similarly, a treatment may be less likely to work if we question its effectiveness, and it is harder to stick to our healing practices when we question our ability to heal.

If you doubt the power of the mind, remember that medical trials take into account the placebo effect. High-level medical research acknowledges that simply believing that one is getting effective treatment can impact the outcome.

In her eye-opening book, *Mind Over Medicine,* Dr. Lissa Rankin makes a powerful argument for the myriad ways our minds affect our health. She begins the exploration with a roundup of studies of the placebo effect. Some of the studies she reviewed showed that:[2]

> Nearly half of asthma patients experienced symptom relief from a fake inhaler or sham acupuncture.

> Half of people with colitis felt better after placebo treatment.

> As many as 40 percent of infertility patients got pregnant while taking placebo fertility drugs.

Ted J. Kaptchuk is a professor of medicine at Harvard Medical School and an international leader in placebo studies. He explains that neuroimaging studies show that placebo treatments have quantifiable effects on specific brain structures like the prefrontal cortex and the rostral anterior cortex, which are responsible for expectations and sensations, respectively. Placebos have a measurable effect on our minds, which in turn affects our bodies.

While Professor Kaptchuk acknowledges that placebos have not been shown to "shrink tumors," he points out, "Over time, changing one's perceptions changes one's physiology. If you experience less pain, you walk more. When you walk more, your body changes."[3]

Conversely, if you expect more pain, you may feel more pain and be more debilitated as a result. That's because there is also something called a nocebo effect, which is when the mention of possible negative effects of a substance, procedure, or health condition can cause patients or research participants to experience those negative effects. In a trial of aspirin for the treatment of angina, participants who were told about possible gastrointestinal (GI) side effects were six times more likely to drop out due to minor GI symptoms, as compared to participants who were not told about the side effects. Similarly, another study showed that using the word "pain" resulted in subjects reporting more pain than using the phrase "cool sensation."[4]

In our healing work, we want to harness the power of the placebo effect and avoid triggering the powers of the nocebo effect.

So, how does the placebo effect work? How do our expectations impact our body? That's still being studied, but it seems to be a combination of the following things:

> Believing that you are on your way to better health can reduce stress and the negative health impacts associated with stress.

> Being cared for and having hope for recovery or relief can stimulate neurotransmitters like serotonin, dopamine, and endorphins that can help ameliorate symptoms, relieve pain, boost your immune system, and lift your mood.

> Our minds seem to have immeasurable and still poorly understood abilities to direct what happens in the blood, cells, nerves, and organs of our bodies.

In the placebo and nocebo effects, conventional medicine recognizes your mind's power to affect your health. When properly convinced of your body's ability to heal, your mind can help make that healing happen. Let's harness that power.

»»» *For Today* «««

Notice how you feel about the placebo effect. Are you excited to explore that power, or are you already wondering if you're too pessimistic for this stuff and if it really makes a difference at all? If you're experiencing any of the latter, explore where that cynicism comes from and how it is serving you, or not.

)(

Day 43
Become a Wholehearted Optimist

Our greatest weakness lies in giving up. The most certain way to succeed is always to try just one more time.

—Thomas Edison

What are some things that trigger the placebo effect, and how can we use that knowledge? Professor Kaptchuk, the Harvard professor and placebo expert, says that what triggers the placebo effect are likely the ritual of medicine; the doctor-patient relationship; and the compassion, trust, and hope engendered there. The good news is that, in addition to seeing doctors, there are many other ways to increase compassion, trust, and hope in your life and thus increase your confidence that you can heal.

Being a pretty cynical person, I wasn't sure I could develop real hope and trust in my ability to heal. I began asking people in the healing arts for advice on how I might improve my attitude. "You can choose to be more optimistic. It's something you can learn" was the response I got from Peg Baim, the director of the Stress Management and Resiliency Training Program at the Benson-Henry Institute for Mind Body Medicine at Massachusetts General Hospital in Boston, when I took their medical symptom reduction program in 2005. She's right. I learned a great deal from that program about the value of becoming optimistic in promoting my healing and continued exploring the topic for years.

There are several medical studies that demonstrate the positive health impact of being optimistic. A 2009 study by the University of Pittsburgh found that "Women who were optimistic—those who expect good rather than bad things to happen—were 14 percent less likely to die from any cause than pessimists and 30 percent less likely to die from heart disease after eight years of follow up in the study."[5]

That's persuasive stuff, but what really convinced me of the value of becoming an optimist were other studies that explained some of why being an optimist is such a powerful tool in getting and staying healthy. In the studies, the optimists reported less disappointment and frustration when they failed at a given task, even though they had expected success more than the pessimists had. To paraphrase the optimists' response: "Too bad. It will probably go better next time." The pessimists tended to feel that the failure confirmed their fears about their abilities and bad luck. As a result, the optimists were more resilient and willing to try again, whereas the pessimists were scared off.[6]

That study was an elegant illustration of how we create our own reality. I realized that I had lived by "Don't get your hopes up" for too long and resisted becoming more optimistic for fear of being disappointed. I became determined to cultivate a more optimistic attitude toward life. I wanted to look forward to the next challenge instead of fearing the next failure. That was a good thing because overcoming a health condition often involves a lot of challenges and some spectacular failures along the way.

In exploring Practice 1, Take Charge, we looked at resistance to change. You may be experiencing some of that resistance right now. "What do you mean, 'Become an optimist'? That's like saying become a foot taller. I am who I am. I can't change that."

If that is the case, I want you to know that I did not come by my optimism muscles easily. I am, by nature and nurture, a pretty dark person. I am cynical. I like my humor burnt-toast dark. On top of that cynical nature, when I was sick, my oldest brother was debilitated by chronic fatigue syndrome. (Thankfully, he, too, has turned his health around.) Then, in the second year of my illness, my father died from a shockingly aggressive form of pulmonary sarcoidosis, which basically means his lungs stopped working. So, in addition to my natural skepticism, my head was full of messages that I had bad genes and, as a result, would just need to get used to being sick for the rest of my life.

But I was lucky. I found teachers and healers who believed I could heal and ingrained the importance of developing optimism in me. Then I used the practices outlined this month to follow through. If I can do it, you can too.

>>> *For Today* <<<

How optimistic are you? What stops you from being more optimistic about your health? What could you do to challenge those attitudes or beliefs that are getting in the way of being more optimistic?

><

Day 44
Christina's Story: Confidence in My Recovery

You gain strength, courage, and confidence by every experience in which you really stop to look fear in the face. You are able to say to yourself, "I have lived through this horror. I can take the next thing that comes along." You must do the thing you think you cannot do.

—Eleanor Roosevelt

Often we need to believe in our ability to heal even more than everyone around us. By instinct and by decision, that is what Christina Hardy did after a traumatic brain injury shattered her reality when she was 29.

After a 1998 car accident in which the car's roof collapsed onto her head, Christina spent three weeks in a coma with little chance of survival. Doctors saved her life by performing a craniotomy: drilling a hole in her skull to relieve massive hemorrhaging.

Christina had a bachelor's in chemistry, had a pilot's license, loved skydiving, and worked as an executive for a computer company. At the time of the crash, she was on vacation in Mexico with her husband. "I had a great life. I had been successful at a lot of things," she recalls.

When Christina woke up from the coma, she couldn't remember who she was. She didn't know how to walk, brush her teeth, or speak English. The left side of her body was paralyzed and her lungs had collapsed. For weeks, she spoke only French, a language she had studied in high school. Each day, when her mother came to visit, she asked the nurses who the "nice lady" was.

Now a divorced mother of two and a yoga practitioner with a talent for glassblowing, Christina has no memory of that harrowing time when doctors predicted she would never walk again and would only minimally recover.

From the start, Christina worked hard. She attributes this drive to a basic human instinct for survival, powered by her long-standing trait of achieving against all odds.

Initially, eight different occupational and cognitive therapists worked with her so she could regain normal life skills. Inspired by a long-term vision of full recovery, she made it happen one small step at a time, using manageable daily goals.

When she began to walk again, she consciously told her legs to move and often fell. The ability to walk without falling became one of the many markers that propelled her forward. "I took every challenge as a competition with my injured, damaged self, and I celebrated every incremental improvement, every small step towards healing as a sign that I could win—a sign that I would get back to a life where my brain injury was not the center and did not dictate what I had to do and did not limit me from what I wanted to do."

For years after her initial recovery, she would tell people upon their first meeting that she was a "brain-injury survivor." But she has so improved that she has stopped feeling the need to do that now.

Physically, she has recovered. Her cognitive abilities, though, remain her greatest challenge. "I work on recovery, like, all the time. It is not a real choice." For example, her language skills returned, but not her math skills, in spite of her previous expertise. "I keep trying to relearn the multiplication tables, but they will not stick."

She also has difficulty with memory and uses systems to help her, such as making sure that everything has a place and keeping items in those places. Her love of art and interest in glassblowing, an interest she initially had as a child—but then forgot and picked up again after the accident— has been useful because it helps focus her mind.

Although Christina has not fully recovered, she has achieved things far beyond her doctors' initial expectations. As she puts it, "I am going to be slugging away at this for the rest of my life and it will make my life interesting."[7]

>»> *For Today* «<«
What can you learn from Christina's experience about setting
health goals, believing in them, and working toward them?

)(

Day 45
Jump In: Choosing Optimism

Buttercup: We'll never survive!
*Westley: Nonsense. You're only saying that because no one
ever has.*

—William Goldman, *The Princess Bride*

Many of us have some resistance to becoming more optimistic. We are
afraid to let our guard down, to be disappointed or disappoint others, or
to change our personality. Those fears can be clues to obstacles to healing:
They point to old beliefs that may be getting in your way. To help unearth
those, try the following exercise.

> **Step 1.** Complete the following sentences. If you can repeat
> this exercise every day for a week (or longer), you will get
> deeper and deeper answers.
>
> • I am afraid that if I become an optimist, I will….
> • I am excited that if I become an optimist, I will….
>
> **Step 2.** You may have old ideas about optimism or optimistic
> people that are getting in the way of becoming optimistic.
> So, answer these questions in as much detail as you can to
> explore those and free you up:
>
> • When you imagine becoming more optimistic, what
>   person, memory, or image comes to mind? (It could be a
>   person or story from your past or from TV, movies, and
>   books; or it could just be a vague impression.)
> • What beliefs about being optimistic did that image or
>   memory instill in you?
> • Do those beliefs still serve you?

- How will those beliefs help or hinder your progress toward healing?

><

Day 46
Surround Yourself With Positive People

When you are seeking to bring big plans to fruition, it is important with whom you regularly associate. Hang out with friends who are like-minded and who are also designing purpose-filled lives. Similarly, be that kind of friend for your friends.

—Mark Twain

To bolster your budding optimism, it's important to find healers, friends, and others who share your confidence. When your belief wavers, they can remind you of all the wonderful possibilities that exist.

Several people helped me immensely by showing unwavering confidence in my ability to heal.

One was my dear friend and teacher Jaye, who had survived kidney failure, dialysis, a kidney transplant, and a series of infections, and outlived a terminal cancer diagnosis by a few years. She had some experience with fearing the worst and overcoming it. The first time she heard my story, she looked at me and said with complete certainty, "You are going to kick this. You are not going to be sick for the rest of your life." When I heard the confidence in her voice, I cried and cried out my fears, and a little bit of her certainty seeped in.

Another person who helped instill confidence in me was Dr. Glenn Rothfeld, the founder of the Rothfeld Center for Integrative Medicine in Arlington, Massachusetts. He let me know that he both understood how sick I was and still felt certain that I could heal completely. His commitment to sticking with me and testing every option until we found a diagnosis and treatment made a huge difference in my ability to believe in a healthy future.

On the days when I doubted that I would ever be able to work or join in on family vacations again, I could borrow some certainty from these and other positive supports in my life to keep me going.

Just as important as surrounding yourself with positive energy is protecting yourself from people—well-meaning or otherwise—with a different attitude. The reality is that many of the people in our lives simply have no clue how to support a person overcoming a serious health challenge. So, if any of the people around you are less than fully positive about your healing potential, or are unhelpfully critical of your self-care decisions, you have several choices. You can:

1. Teach them to be more positive.

2. Ask them to keep their mouth shut. (I find that putting my hand, palm out, right up in their face works well when necessary.)

3. Ignore them.

4. Avoid discussing your health with them.

It is hard to keep up your own confidence when others are tearing it down. Don't let people do that to you.

>>> *For Today* <<<

List some people who have voiced confidence in your ability to heal. If appropriate, contact them to tell them that you appreciate it, encourage them to do it more, and ask them to share their confidence with other friends, family members, and your healthcare providers.

)(

Day 47
Integrate Useful Feedback

You know how advice is. You only want it if it agrees with what you wanted to do anyway.

—John Steinbeck

Yesterday we talked about protecting yourself from people who don't share your confident attitude about your healing. The trick is we need to balance that with maintaining an openness to feedback.

That raises the question: Which feedback should you listen to? You may get a lot. When people hear you have a health challenge, it's suddenly open season for unsolicited advice: "I've heard those drugs are terrible for you." "Blue-green algae saved my husband's cousin." "An osteopath? Is that a real doctor?"

Somewhere in that onslaught of well-intentioned, but potentially annoying, advice could be some good perspectives to consider. Although anybody might have good insights to share, someone's advice is more likely to be helpful if she has taken the time to understand your circumstances and options. Others who are just stating opinions based on their own experience and biases are less likely to have relevant information to share.

Having said that, I have learned to almost never rule things out entirely. It's helpful to file ideas away for the future. Some advice that feels thoughtless or irrelevant at the time may actually be a useful perspective that you just aren't ready for yet. Put some things away to pull out later and explore with your healthcare providers if you find that your current approach isn't working.

There were many things that I initially heard as annoying, unsolicited advice that turned out to be key to getting my life back: "Your diet isn't working. You need a more hard-core detoxifying diet if you want to heal." "You have to quit working and get help in the house if you ever want to get better." I'm glad that I kept those pieces of advice on the back burner to return to when I needed them.

>>> *For Today* <<<
What disregarded advice have you gotten in the past that might move you forward in your healing now?

><

Day 48
Cultivate Trust

The function of prayer is not to influence God, but rather to change the nature of the one who prays.

—Søren Kierkegaard

As we explore how to become more optimistic, it's important to address the question of how to integrate the reality that bad things do happen into a sense of optimism. I've found that the most optimistic people bolster their confidence in the future with a deep sense of trust.

According to one understanding of *Mussar*, the Jewish path to ethical and spiritual growth, trust (or *bitachon* in Hebrew) means trusting in God that all is good *right now*, even when it doesn't seem that way. Full disclosure: I'm not there yet. I'm guessing you might not be, either. If a friend is dying of cancer or there is a war going on, I struggle to accept that it is okay and part of a larger, divine plan that I just can't see. But I do aspire to develop more of that sense of mystery because I know it can help me move through the world with more optimism and less fear.

For those of us who are not fully enlightened *Mussar* practitioners, here are some beginner levels of trust where we can start:

> › Even when things do not appear to be for the good, they may be for the good eventually.

> › Even if things do not turn out as we want, between our own resources and the support of the Divine, nature, and those around us, we have what we need to get through anything.

The two stories that follow should help to discern what that really means.

The Donation

The director of an antipoverty organization spent an entire year convincing a philanthropist to donate $85,000 to his organization so he could build a new computer lab for vocational training. After a year of negotiating, it seemed like the deal was sealed. That's when the philanthropist withdrew with no explanation. The organization director was a religious man and, instead of railing against the philanthropist, his immediate response was "Thank God!" He explained clearly that the donor was not the right person to establish this important program and that the right person would come along soon. Two weeks later, an elderly woman who admired the organization's work passed away and left the organization $80,000.

I was the fund-raising consultant who had been partially responsible for setting up the original $85,000 donation. Suffice to say that my reaction was not "Thank God!" when I heard the donor had backed out. It was something far less printable here. The director's reaction rocked my world. How different would my life be if I could respond to every seeming setback with "Thank God!" and the faith that through my own hard work and the support of the universe, it would work out in the end? If I could react to every new situation with that sense of trust instead of the anxiety that often ruled my thoughts, my life would be radically different.

The Strange Sabbath

A man once visited a small town on the Sabbath. He had been told that the local synagogue was a friendly place that welcomed guests with honored roles during the service and a delicious lunch afterward. But he was disappointed. Instead of receiving an honor during the service himself, he was ignored, whereas all the honored roles were given to several rough, unkempt men in the back of the synagogue. After the service, several platters of beautiful food were brought out for lunch, but were quickly returned to the kitchen, and the man was offered nothing to eat.

The man was dismayed that the synagogue was so different from what he had expected. He asked a member what was going on and was told, "The men you saw have been falsely imprisoned for years and the congregation has worked hard to free them. We are celebrating their release, which just happened yesterday. We also have a tradition of contributing all the food from our lunch to a home for the elderly once a month. So, on those Sabbaths, we bring the platters out so that we can see what a lovely feast we are sending to them, but we all eat at home instead."[8]

It takes a sense of mystery and a dose of humility to trust that all will be well and that we don't always have the whole picture. That trust, in turn, can enable us to approach every situation with a much more optimistic attitude. From handling rain at a picnic to integrating the news of a serious illness, developing trust enables you to be more expansive and less fearful in every area of your life. It's not an easy shift to make, but it is well worth trying.

>»» *For Today* «««

How much trust do you have in your life? Would you like to develop more? Are you open to developing the sense of mystery and humility it takes to get there? Check out *www.mussarinstitute.org*, and *www.Kirva.org* for more information about *Mussar*.

)(

Day 49
Replace Negative Thoughts With Positive Ones

What you think, you become. What you feel, you attract.
What you imagine, you create.

—Buddha

Today's quote is attributed to Gautama Buddha, the first Buddha, on whose teachings Buddhism was founded. He had some game. We would do well to listen to him on this one. We create an enormous part of our reality and all kinds of self-fulfilling prophecies based on what we think and feel in response to the events in our lives. If we expect to be sick for years, or in pain all week, it is much more likely that will come to pass. Sometimes, we unconsciously create that kind of expectation just by the language we use. To avoid that, for many of us, the first step in healing is to shed our identity as a sick or disabled person.

This may sound like a contradiction to the start of Practice 1, Take Charge, where I wrote about the importance of accepting the reality of our health challenges. Like many aspects of healing, this is a tricky balance. We do need to accept how serious our health challenges are. Here, we are talking about how we think and feel about our health challenges, once we have accepted their (sometimes-harsh) reality. Try these two sentences on for size:

1. I am sick.

2. My strong body is overcoming a health challenge.

I don't know about you, but I am a big fan of the second sentence. I'll tell you why. The first sentence, *I am sick*, does not move you toward healing. It's worth considering dropping that phrase from your thoughts and speech entirely. If you regularly think, *I am sick, I am in pain*, or *I am fat*, then being sick, in pain, or overweight becomes an integral part of your identity. As a result, you may unconsciously make choices that perpetuate that reality because we are all resistant to losing integral parts of our identity, even if we don't like them.

In contrast, the second sentence, *My strong body is overcoming a health challenge*, can be a powerful tool in promoting health. First, it's positive, which is useful when you are trying to cultivate a positive attitude. Second, it reminds you of the reality that, given the right nutrition, rest, and exercise, your body has remarkable healing abilities. Last, it describes your current situation as changing and fluid, which is true of any life circumstance. Rather than trapping yourself with a static label, it envisions you growing and changing in new directions.

Try saying each of these phrases, or similar ones that are a better match for your circumstances, and see the difference in how they make you feel. Starting today, try incorporating a more positive, dynamic version of what's going on with your body into your thoughts and repeat it often. What you say in the privacy of your own mind becomes what you believe. Wouldn't you rather believe that you have a strong body and are overcoming a health challenge than that you are just...sick?

Although we don't fully understand the power of the mind to impact the body, it is clear that we would do well to ensure that, whatever impact our own mind has on our body, it is in the healing direction that we seek.

>>> *For Today* <<<

What are some ways that you identify yourself or your health status that could be jiggled a bit to be more positive and take into account the fluid, changing reality you are in?

)(

Day 50
Notice Your Inner Critic

There is nothing either good or bad, but thinking makes it so.

—Shakespeare

Using more positive and dynamic language to talk about your health status can help you feel immensely more confident about your healing work. You still, though, have to contend with your inner critic. There are many names for that voice in your head that can berate you and sabotage ambitious projects. The inner critic, the anxious chatterbox, and the sh*tty committee are just some. There are variations in frequency, message, and volume, but we all have one.

I'm not talking about a wise guide that constructively tells us when we are a bit off course. I am talking about a nasty voice made up of messages that we internalized when we were young. Some highlights might include: "You can't do that." "Why can't you get your act together?" or "Be good or else!"

We originally received these messages from authority figures like parents, teachers, coaches, and religious leaders, or from the media and larger society. They usually came from people who meant well, in misguided efforts to improve our behavior. Sometimes they weren't even said to us, but to someone we loved and we internalized them just the same. Other times the messages weren't said directly at all, but we inferred them from what we saw around us. Often, we received these limiting messages as part of the experience of being targeted by sexism, racism, homophobia, ableism, or other prejudices.

However we received the messages, it may have felt or actually been necessary to heed them when we were young to feel safe in the world or to please the adults around us. Today, that negative voice is only harmful. Learning how to tame it and even transform it into a source for support can make a world of difference in your ability to believe in a better future and in your own capacity to get there.

The first step to transforming that voice is to notice when it is happening. Sometimes it is a very clear thought like "There is no way I can do this. I am crazy to even try." In those cases, rather than accepting it at face value, you can take a moment, switch it to second person: "There is no way you can do this. You are crazy to even try," and notice how you would feel if a friend or loved one talked to you that way. Pretty mad, right? Notice that feeling and determine that if you wouldn't let others speak to you that way, you won't do it to yourself.

Sometimes it is less clear that your inner critic is sabotaging your efforts. If you are feeling drawn to unhealthy habits or addictions, it's a good indicator that the inner critic is on the prowl. Rachel Eddins, the founder of Eddins Counseling in Houston, Texas, and main author of a fabulous blog at *www.eddinscounseling.com*, describes how giving into your addictions can be a clear sign that you are being impacted by those old, negative messages. She explains: "...this type of communication is anxiety-provoking and shaming, which is the opposite of motivation. It triggers us to avoid, reduce anxiety and stay safe…Avoidance generally includes things such as procrastination, addictive behaviors (such as overeating, grazing when not hungry, drinking, smoking); behaviors such as constantly checking your smartphone, or watching excessive TV…"[9]

As I write this book, when I feel a pull to surf the Internet or snack when I'm not hungry, I know that my inner critic is acting up. Even though I can't hear it clearly, I know that the anxious, antsy feeling I sometimes get comes from subconscious messages that my writing isn't good enough or this is all a waste of time. To escape those messages and the anxiety they stir up, I suddenly feel a powerful urge to eat a PB&J sandwich or watch Jennifer Lawrence interviews on YouTube. This urge arises intermittently all day long when I'm writing. I'm lucky that my addictions run to things like childhood lunch items and stories about empowered female celebrities, instead of liquor or hard drugs; otherwise I would be in trouble. I am serious about that. We all have addictions. Some of us are just fortunate enough to have ones that are not life-threatening.

The same thing can happen when you try to exercise, prepare healthy meals, or do any other self-care practice. Old, negative messages about your body, your health, or your abilities can pop up without even being fully verbalized. They just manifest as an intangible sense of anxiety or malaise, followed by a strong urge to turn to work, food, shopping, alcohol, drugs, cigarettes, the Internet, or any other number of distractions to escape. Does this sound familiar? What's your distraction of choice?

»»» For Today ««

Practice noticing when your inner critic is kicking in, either as a clear voice or as a less-conscious pull to distract yourself. Notice what your distractions are and, instead of giving into them, give yourself a moment to notice the uncomfortable feelings driving you to escape in the first place. Then, take a moment to tell yourself that those feelings come from old, useless messages, and it's best not to take them seriously. If necessary, tell a friend about your effort and get support to win this battle.

)(

Day 51
Kick the Negativity Habit

You need to learn how to select your thoughts just the same way you select your clothes every day.

—Elizabeth Gilbert

Another way to transform the tide of negative messages from your inner critic is to take any negative thought that pops into your head and turn it into a positive affirmation. Without thinking about it or arguing with it, you can just flip it to serve you. Old messages and beliefs like "I am undisciplined" work, at best, as unconscious blocks to making the changes you need to get healthier and, at worst, fully conscious excuses for not even trying to make the changes. You can replace them with thoughts and beliefs that support your healing like "I'm disciplined and able to achieve my goals." It's not easy, but you can do it.

We now know that habitual thoughts and actions create neural pathways in our brains, like well-worn ruts in a road that our thoughts repeatedly follow over and over again. We also know that, though it takes time, those neural pathways can be adjusted with time. It requires creating new ruts in the road. The best way to do that is to constantly offer your mind positive thoughts to replace your negative ones.

These positive affirmations may not feel true at first. But they are. In any area that is a challenge for you, I promise you, no matter how much of a basket case you think you are, there are some elements you do have under control. You may think of yourself as disorganized, but there are ways in which you are organized, even if it is just that you remember to brush your teeth or make it to work most days. So focus on that. It is not all black-and-white. What we focus on grows. Let's focus on the good stuff.

>>> *For Today* <<<

Notice what negative thoughts consistently pop into your head and how they make you feel.

)(

Day 52
Jump In: Flip Your Negative Thoughts

"Of course there must be lots of Magic in the world," he said wisely one day, "but people don't know what it is like or how to make it. Perhaps the beginning is just to say nice things are going to happen until you make them happen."

—Frances Hodgson Burnett

Step 1. Think of several negative phrases that your inner critic tends to throw at you and write them each down.

Step 2. Flip each negative message and create a positive affirmation instead.

Here are some examples:

NEGATIVE	POSITIVE
I can't live without sugar.	I don't need sugar. I eat healing food that nourishes my body.
I am undisciplined.	I am disciplined. I have a powerful mind.
There is no way out of this situation.	I can get help and figure this out. The possibilities are endless.

Step 3. Practice doing this throughout the day. Any time that you sense an old negative thought running through your head, flip it into a positive affirmation and repeat that to yourself instead.

><

Might this previous exercise feel a bit hokey? Yes. Is it useful? Very. Although I do understand if you are having a "too cool for school" moment, it's a good idea to get over that. A lot of cool people have used this stuff with great success. Do whatever you can to get comfortable with this practice of switching negative thoughts to positive ones throughout the day until it becomes a habit. It has immense potential to help you achieve your health goals and all your other goals as well.

Day 53
Jump In: Fire Your Inner Critic

It's not what you say out of your mouth that determines your life. It's what you whisper to yourself that has the most power.

—Robert T. Kiyosaki

This is an adapted and summarized version of a powerfully liberating exercise I first encountered 20 years ago in Robert Gerzon's program "Mastering Anxiety," which he developed for the Harvard Community Health Plan. You can read more about these ideas in Gerzon's insightful book, *Finding Serenity in the Age of Anxiety.*

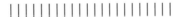

Step 1: Think again about all the mean things that your inner critic has said to you in the last week and notice how damaging and hurtful that voice is.

Step 2: Write a termination letter to your inner critic, letting it know that its services are no longer needed. Thank it for the purpose it might have served many, many years ago when it first arrived and let it know that, as of today, it is fired. Make it detailed. Let it know why you don't want its nasty messages anymore and how quickly you want it to pack up and leave.

Step 3: Write a want ad for a new inner voice that is loving, supportive, fair, and thoughtful. Describe the kind of guidance and support you are looking for in an inner voice and the responsibilities it would have. Put that into the advertisement.

Step 4: Notice over the next few days and weeks whenever that inner critic tries to come back into work. Firmly remind it that it was fired and look for the kinder inner voice to offer you support and guidance instead. Re-read your termination letter and want ad a few times if that helps.

><

Day 54
Make Stress Work for You

I was a little excited but mostly blorft. "Blorft" is an adjective I just made up that means "Completely overwhelmed but proceeding as if everything is fine and reacting to the stress with the torpor of a possum." I have been blorft every day for the past seven years.

—Tina Fey

It can be very tough to keep building your confidence and trust when you are dealing with a situation as potentially stressful as a significant health condition. In addition, health experts from the Mayo Clinic to the Centers for Disease Control confirm that stress can be bad for your health.[10, 11] Yet, it's not that simple. Stress is neither good nor bad. It is just part of life. How we perceive and react to stress and how long it goes on uninterrupted is what gives it the power to derail us both emotionally and physically.

For the next few days, let's focus on how you can be in a potentially stressful situation—like dealing with a significant health challenge—without being derailed by the negative stress it could induce. In fact, I want to offer the possibility that you could even learn to be exhilarated by the growth challenges it offers. I know. I just crossed several lines of decency by suggesting that you embrace your MS, cancer, infertility, diabetes, or chronic Lyme disease as an exhilarating challenge. I'm not saying that you don't also get to be furious that you have to deal with it in the first place. Being able to hold both feelings simultaneously is a key to all this work. Bear with me, keep an open mind, and let's see where this goes.

As you probably know, the stress response is the fight-or-flight response triggered when you perceive something as threatening. Hormones like adrenaline and cortisol are released and cause a number of physiological changes, including increased blood sugar, blood pressure and heart rate, and a suppressed immune response and digestive system. The stress response can be extremely helpful by keeping you temporarily alert, focused, and energetic in times of need, especially when it recedes quickly after it is no longer necessary. However, when it is triggered repeatedly over the long term, it can wreak havoc with your emotional and physical well-being.

It's important to notice two things about the stress response. First, it is triggered when you *perceive* something as threatening. That means that changing your perception can affect how stressed you feel. The second is that short periods of experiencing the stress response are not necessarily bad for you and can even be beneficial. So, figuring out how to make the most of your stress response and then limit the amount of time that you are stuck in it are two key ways to manage stress.

Knowing all that, there is a lot you can do to change how you relate to potentially stressful circumstances in your life and how much emotional stress you carry around as a result. That will keep you healthier and make it easier to feel confident about your health goals in the long run.

>>> *For Today* <<<
Notice what's causing you to feel stressed in your life today. How willing are you to entertain the notion that experiencing stress does not have to be bad for you?

)(

Day 55
Choose Your Response to Stress

The greatest weapon against stress is our ability to choose one thought over another.

—William James

Stressful events are in the eye of the beholder. One person's fantasy could be another's stress extravaganza. Take public speaking. Someone who enjoys public speaking experiences the stress of preparing and giving her speech as exhilarating and challenging, with a dollop of fear. It may trigger the stress response, but only temporarily and in moderation.

Someone who is terrified of public speaking, on the other hand, may experience her stress response kicking in weeks before the event itself as she fearfully anticipates it. She experiences the stress of the situation as a very negative thing, and has significant anxiety and emotional and physical stress for a long period as a result.

It's not quite the same with health challenges. I don't expect anyone to immediately respond to a stressor like a type 2 diabetes diagnosis with enthusiasm and excitement. There is, though, a continuum. Imagine someone at one end of the continuum who catastrophizes that diagnosis, imagines the worst possible outcomes, and can't begin to envision a life with less sugar and more vegetables. On the other end of the spectrum we might find someone who is deeply upset by the diagnosis, but can also work up enthusiasm for taking on a new diet and exercise regime and finally getting healthy for real. The first person's level of emotional stress will be much higher and cause significant physical and emotional hardship. What is the difference between these two people?

Dr. Susan Krauss Whitbourne, a professor of psychology and the author of *The Search for Fulfillment*, says that "You only feel stressed when you believe that you lack the resources to manage a threat or challenge. If you think your coping abilities are up to snuff, then you'll be fine."[12]

That's such an important message. If you set up good support for yourself, educate yourself, develop a positive mind set, and commit to working toward a good outcome, you will feel better about your abilities to succeed and be able to experience any event as less stressful and upsetting. You can change how potentially stressful situations affect you by how prepared you feel to deal with them.

Another way you can change how stress impacts you is by avoiding double-dipping. That is the term coined by a friend of mine for when you're not just stressed, but you're also stressed out about being stressed. Research shows that's not good for you. A Yale psychologist, Alia Crum, and her team found that whether people viewed stress negatively or positively affected how stress impacted them. If they thought stress was bad for them and got stressed out by being stressed (double-dipping), they were worse off than if they perceived stress to be a good thing.[13]

The 2013 study looked at two groups of people. The first group believed that stress was energy-sapping, potentially harmful, and something to be avoided, whereas the second group viewed stress as performance-enhancing, growth-inducing, and something to be sought out. The study found that the "[i]ndividuals who endorse a stress-is-enhancing mindset reported having better health than those who endorse a stress-is-debilitating mindset: specifically, respondents reported fewer symptoms of depression and anxiety while also reporting higher levels of energy."[14]

That's amazing. If you go through a stressful experience, but you think it is good for you, you are significantly protected from many of the negative impacts of stress. You'll experience fewer of the negative effects and more of the positive ones.

It makes the next steps pretty clear, right? Dealing with a significant health condition inherently carries some stress with it. It might be a good idea to do whatever you can to convince yourself that stress can be your friend.

>>> *For Today* <<<

Explore these themes to help you internalize this idea of stress as a potentially positive force for growth. You can also watch a fabulous Ted Talk on YouTube called "How to Make Stress Your Friend" by Kelly McGonigal, the author of *The Upside of Stress*, or search *benefits of stress* online.

)(

Day 56
De-Stress Your Life

Businessman on the phone, looking at a calendar: "No. Thursday's out. How about never—is never good for you?"
—Bob Mankoff, *New Yorker* cartoon

Let's do a quick review of two ideas we've explored so far about stress:

1. Feeling like you have enough resources to meet a challenge can reduce your negative reaction to stress.

2. Smaller amounts of stress are less likely to cause you emotional and physical harm than longer-term stress.

It can be a challenge to put these ideas to work for you because: 1) When you have been dealing with a significant health challenge for a long time, all your resources can feel depleted, and 2) many health conditions are long-term situations that dole out stress on a regular basis.

One way to address both of these challenges is to prioritize—to cut out any unnecessary stressors in your life in order to focus your mental and physical resources on your healing work. Real healing work can be a part- to full-time job. Trying to squeeze it in between all your other responsibilities can be very stressful. If any of those other responsibilities can be considered optional, do whatever you can to get rid of them. (If you have had a long-term health challenge for years, you may have already had to shed many things and this may not be your issue.)

I have seen a woman with small children with a two-months-to-live cancer prognosis struggle to give up a part-time fund-raising job to focus on her health and family. I have seen mothers with chronic fatigue syndrome insist on preparing all their family's home-cooked meals rather than simplify or outsource child- and house-care to take care of themselves. We've all witnessed men with heart disease who would rather cut off their arm than cut back their work hours. As we discussed in the previous section, there are all kinds of emotional and logistical reasons why people struggle to give up some of their responsibilities and focus on their health situation. These are not simple decisions to make. But cutting back is sometimes the key to moving forward.

>>> *For Today* <<<
Begin exploring where you might be able to cut back to decrease the stress on your system and shift more resources to your healing efforts. What prevents you from cutting back? What are you afraid of? Are those fears worth listening to?

✕

Day 57
Jump In: Prioritize Your Life

> *[Steve] Jobs insisted that Apple focus on just two or three priorities at a time. "There is no one better at*

turning off the noise that is going on around him,"
Tim Cook [then Apple's Chief Operating Officer] said.
"That allows him to focus on a few things and say no to
many things. Few people are really good at that."

—Walter Isaacson

This exercise is designed to help you prioritize what is truly important as you work to heal and to identify activities that may not be serving you right now.

Step 1. List all the major things in your life that are taking your time these days. This could include a job, a volunteer position, parenting, responsibilities you have in your family, a hobby that you are committed to, a self-care practice, or anything else that takes your time and energy.

Step 2. Ask yourself the following four questions about each item:

1. Is this moving me forward in my healing process?

2. If the answer to #1 is *no*, is it absolutely necessary to do this thing for some other reason?

3. Can this item either be jettisoned entirely or possibly done by somebody else?

4. If you had no audience, nobody to disappoint or impress, would you still answer the previous questions the same way?

Step 3. If the answers to any of the previous questions were *no*, explore if and how you can cut out or reduce that activity from your life, even temporarily, to give you more time and energy to focus on your healing with less stress.

)(

Day 58
Discover the Relaxation Response

It's not the load that breaks you down. It's the way you carry it.

—Lou Holtz

Given life's realities, even after you've eliminated the unnecessary demands in your life and decided to feel more enthusiastic about taking on the challenges of the remaining ones, you will still experience some stress now and then. In fact, if you are dealing with a serious health condition, you may still experience a lot. Let's look at one more way to help you become more resilient to the negative impacts of stress: the relaxation response.

The term *relaxation response* was coined by Dr. Herbert Benson of Harvard Medical School in 1974 and is "a state of relaxed, passive attention to a repetitive or absorbing stimulus that turns off the inner dialogue, thereby decreasing arousal of the sympathetic nervous system."[15]

As the physical opposite of the fight-or-flight response, the relaxation response relaxes your muscles, lowers your heart rate, decreases negative emotions and their associated stress hormones, and increases positive emotions and their associated hormones. If elicited regularly, it can interrupt a chronic state of stress and give your body and mind a relaxed "home base" to return to.

Michael, a 50-year-old with chronic back pain, says that before he figured out how to integrate the relaxation response regularly into his life, even when he was supposedly at rest, his mind was still going a million miles an hour with worries and anxiety. He felt like he never got a break. Once he learned to be more mindful and slow things down occasionally, it gave him a sense of what it felt like to escape all that for a bit and just be. Now he has a state he can return to whenever he needs it, to take the edge off and help him manage his pain. By developing that more relaxed home base, even doing it only five or 15 minutes every day can have a big impact on your mood.

That sounds pretty good, right? It would be great to escape from the chronic fight-or-flight mode and teach your body and mind to chill out a bit. How do you do that?

The most obvious way to achieve the relaxed, passive attention necessary to elicit the relaxation response is to meditate. Studies have been done on the myriad health benefits of meditating, showing that it can help reduce blood pressure; symptoms of irritable bowel syndrome; anxiety and depression; insomnia, and the duration and severity of acute respiratory illness.[16]

One of the things that I learned in the 12-week Medical Symptom Reduction Program at the Benson-Henry Institute for Mind Body Medicine in Boston was that, in addition to traditional seated meditation, there are several other ways one can elicit the relaxation response. Let's take a look tomorrow.

>>> *For Today* <<<

Take 15 minutes to pick up your old meditation practice again or listen to a guided relaxation or meditation program online. You could also take some time to search the phrase *relaxation response* online.

><

Day 59
Practice the Relaxation Response

Half an hour's meditation each day is essential, except when you are busy. Then a full hour is needed.

—St. Francis de Sales

Here are a number of ways to elicit the relaxation response. The main ingredients are focused attention on something pleasant and relaxed breathing.

Meditation

Meditation can sound intimidating or off-putting if you haven't explored it before. In fact, the basics are just sitting and breathing in a relaxed manner while focusing on something pleasant, or at least benign. If you have had a meditation practice in the past, this would be a good time to dive back in. If not, look at local wellness providers or adult-education centers for meditation classes or find a guided-meditation recording online. Guided meditations often go through a simple muscle-relaxation exercise or a visioning exercise of something pleasant. I confess that I have found meditation difficult at times. On my own, I tend to go to town on the to-do list in my head, worry about the future, or fall fast asleep. Using guided meditations helps me stay focused and relax.

You can purchase excellent guided meditation recordings online from the Benson-Henry Institute for Mind Body Medicine or download free ones from the UCLA Mindful Awareness Research Center.[17]

Walking Meditation

Walk slowly around your block or even just in your house. You can count your steps, notice how your arms and legs move, or count how many red things you see along the way—anything to give you something benign on which to focus. If your mind begins running away with an idea and pulls you from your relaxed focus, one option is to imagine placing that thought in a bag and leaving it on the side of your path as you continue along the way.

Prayer and Gratitude

Rather than trying to empty one's mind, for many people, repeating memorized prayers of gratitude and praise or just speaking out thoughts and ideas to the Divine can be a deeply meditative activity. Alternatively, you can choose to list three to five things that you are grateful for and take a minute to focus on the details of each one, really internalizing the sense of gratitude they give you and letting other worries fall away.

Yoga, Qigong, and Tai Chi

Different types of yoga are more or less meditative, but there are a wide variety of classes and videos that give you the kind of relaxed breathing and focused attention that can elicit the relaxation response. Don't give up if you don't like the first one you try.

Qigong and Tai Chi are two forms of gentle martial arts. They can be very meditative and, like yoga, have the added benefit of improving strength and flexibility.

Music, Song, and Dance

Sometimes just having music to focus on instead of sitting in a silent room can help sustain your focus and relax your mind. More specifically, singing with a relaxed, sustained focus on the lyrics and music, while letting other thoughts drop away, can be a very meditative experience. Like singing, dancing with a focus on the music and an intent to let go of other thoughts can be liberating and relaxing at the same time.

Breath

One of the most useful things I learned at the Benson-Henry Institute for Mind Body Medicine was the power of the breath. We were encouraged to do a "mini" anytime we needed it. A mini is just taking a deep, relaxed breath into your diaphragm, holding the breath for a few seconds, and then letting it out slowly as you relax the muscles in your face, neck, shoulders, and chest. It's a remarkably powerful way to reset your nervous system and keep stress at bay. I've used it several times to deflect stress about my writing as I created today's entry. It makes a world of difference.

>»> *For Today* «<«

Pick the method of eliciting the relaxation response that most appeals to you or that you think you will most likely use this week. Write down anything that you need to organize, download, borrow, or purchase to try out that practice. Make an appointment with yourself in your calendar to try it out as many times as makes sense for you this week. Even five to 15 minutes can make a difference.

)(

Day 60
Imagine a Fabulous Future

I visualize exactly how I am going to pitch to each hitter and I see and feel myself throwing exactly the pitches that I want to throw. Before I ever begin to warm up at the ballpark, I've faced all of the opposition's hitters four times and I've gotten my body ready for exactly what it is I want to do.

—Nolan Ryan

Now that you've begun to decrease and manage the stress in your current life, let's turn to creating your future. You may have heard of using visualizing—imagining positive outcomes in your mind—to shape your future. The first place I came across it was in the course I took at the Benson-Henry Institute for Mind Body Medicine.

We watched a short video about an elite track runner who had hit a plateau in his training; he wasn't able to improve his speed the way he wanted to. His coach saw that he was holding a lot of tension when he ran and began using intensive visualizing with him. He had the runner repeatedly watch a film of a cheetah running (needless to say, the cheetah was not tense when it ran) and taught him visualizing techniques to conjure up the cheetah image as often as he could all day long. The runner did this for some significant amount of time. You've probably guessed the outcome already. The runner improved his race times and, even more impressively, looked different in the before-and-after videos of his running. He actually looked less tense and more fluid—like a cheetah.

I received two lessons from this inspirational video. First: Visualizing can truly change what our bodies are capable of doing. Second: Smart, practical people with big ambitions use it to meet their goals—and, hey, I want to be a smart person who meets her goals, too.

Today and tomorrow I want to share two powerful visualizing tools that can help you make your healthier future more concrete. The first is a vision board. To make one, you collect images, words, and phrases that represent how you want your life to be and put them all together. You can do it by cutting and pasting photos on your computer or by putting a combination of magazine images, your own photos, and computer images on a piece of poster board. Then post it somewhere that you will see it regularly and use it as inspiration to motivate you to do the self-care work.

As you create inspiring visualizations for yourself, keep in mind that it's also helpful to include images of what it will take to get there, like researching treatments, eating healthy meals, exercising, meditating, or bringing in more support.

Pauline, who is 35 and has MS, made a vision board a few years ago. She says that looking at it now is both heartbreaking, as she remembers how much worse off she used to be, and incredibly moving, as she notices how far she's come. Her vision board contained many images of playing outdoors—at the beach or in the woods. When she made the board, those seemed like unattainable dreams for her and now, though she still has physical challenges, she is able to get out and enjoy the outdoors regularly. Having that vision and fighting hard for it were big parts of what enabled her to make that progress.

Get some poster board and magazines, and look online for images that inspire you. Then begin to create your own vision board of how you'd like your life to look. For more details on how to create a vision board and its benefits, download the free guide "Create Your Vision Board" at *www. EverydayHealingforYou.com/tools.*

)(

Day 61
Jump In: Use Visualization to Turbo-Charge Your Healing

Alice laughed: "There's no use trying," she said; "one can't believe impossible things."

"I daresay you haven't had much practice," said the Queen. "When I was younger, I always did it for half an hour a day. Why, sometimes I've believed as many as six impossible things before breakfast."

—Lewis Carroll

Alissa Cohen's fantastic book, *Living on Live Food*, has a powerful section on visualizing to achieve your goals. She talks about the importance of setting a few clear, tangible goals and coming up with short, affirming descriptions of them that you can say to yourself and envision several times a day. She encourages readers to write the goals in just a few words and in the present tense. If we envision things as happening off in the future, they may always remain there.

Some examples might be:

> "I exercise vigorously."

> "I enjoy fun-filled family vacations."

> "I counsel effectively and lucratively."

> "I dance ecstatically and pain-free."

> "I live joyfully."

We know that goals help us keep moving forward with real momentum. Using your imagination to visualize these goals adds more force to that momentum. The more that you "see" something regularly and in detail, the more you believe it can be true, accept it into your life, and make it a reality. Here is a place where "You have to see it to believe it" really applies.

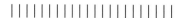

Step 1. Choose three areas in your life (career, family, friends, physical, spiritual, community, financial, etc.) and imagine how you want them each to be. For example, if you are unable to work now, what is your dream job for when your health improves? Or, if you are unable to exercise much, how do you hope to be moving your body in the future? If your social life is limited, how do you want it to look? Be ambitious. Don't be afraid to write what you really want, regardless of how likely you think it is right now.

Step 2. Create a short, descriptive sentence (ideally five or fewer words) to describe how you want each of those three areas of your life to look. See the previous examples.

Step 3. Come up with a mental image, filled with as much detail as possible, to represent each goal—for example, a mental picture of yourself dancing with friends or working passionately with colleagues.

Step 4. Repeat these sentences to yourself one to three times each day and visualize the accompanying images. Choosing specific times in the day to do the visualizations will help you remember. You can do it daily during morning stretching, while doing dishes, or while brushing your teeth. Try to focus on each image for at least a few seconds and ideally closer to a minute—long enough to feel some emotion about it and look forward to doing it.

)(

If you are like most people, including me, when you first start this exercise, the internal conversation may go something like this:

Confident Self: I exercise vigorously.

Doubtful Self: Yeah, right! You exercise your tush muscle vigorously by lying around all day.

Confident Self: I exercise vigorously.

Doubtful Self: Who are you kidding? You haven't been able to exercise vigorously in years and probably never will again.

Confident Self: I exercise vigorously.

Doubtful Self: I just don't want you to be disappointed when this hocus-pocus doesn't work.

Confident Self: I exercise vigorously.

Doubtful Self: Fine. Have it your way.

Confident Self: I exercise vigorously!

The key is not to give up—not to let your inner critic or cynic prevent you from using this powerful tool. It feels more natural with time and becomes easier to believe and eventually—amazingly—it can begin to be true. About one year after I started visualizing my goals regularly, I had vastly improved my health and was exercising regularly, beginning to get back to work again, and living much more joyfully after six years of not being able to do much of anything. It took a lot of hard work and many setbacks on the way. But visualizations like these gave me an incentive to move forward, develop my confidence, and achieve my goals.

Day 62
Be the Awe-Inspiring Hero of Your Own Life

A hero is an ordinary individual who finds the strength to persevere and endure in spite of overwhelming obstacles.

—Christopher Reeve

This tool in strengthening my belief in myself and the goodness of the universe was given to me like a beautiful gift by my husband, David, one evening when I was spending hours every day doing all kinds of self-care in my last (and successful) effort at getting well.

It was hard work. As you know, a serious healing effort to overcome a major health challenge can be very physically, logistically, and emotionally difficult. The only way to slog through the diets, exercise, self-care regimes, pain, or difficult medical treatments is to have absolute confidence that you are worth it and that it will make your life immensely better. I had hit a point where I doubted both. I was feeling overwhelmed by my healing regime and like I was a big loser for having been sick for so long with an undiagnosed illness. Of course, I wasn't a loser and I could handle my healing regime when I got help. It was just hard to remember that. This way of reframing my experience helped immensely.

David came home from work and I was sitting at the kitchen table, lonely and sad. *"Auughh!"* I moaned to him. "I am a loser. I have no life! I have to spend so much more time on my health than everybody else. I have to sleep 10 hours a night. My food takes forever to prepare and I'm still not bringing in any money for our family and can't take care of the kids by myself or go out in the evenings. I spend all of my time just trying to get healthy. Other people don't have to do this. I'm lonely and I hate it!"

It was a pretty pathetic self-pity session and it would have been perfectly reasonable for David to just remind me how lucky I was that I was beginning to get better. But instead he listened for a while, held me as I cried, and then said this: "You are not a loser to me. To me, you are like an elite athlete training for the big event. You need your body to do something amazing, so you are putting yourself through a rigorous training routine to get there. Like an athlete, it takes a ton of discipline because it takes hours of work every day, separates you from your friends for a while, limits what you can eat, and makes you feel lonely. You are focused on a goal. And I have total faith that you are going to win big in your event." When he finished his speech, I wiped my eyes and said, "Really? You don't think I'm a big loser? You think I'm like an elite athlete?" "One hundred percent," he responded.

That was a big turning point. I still sometimes resented the amount of time and energy I had to put into my healing regime, as well as the intense limitations it put on me. But I was able to see it in a much more positive light. I wasn't a pathetic victim. I was a heroic figure because I was choosing to take care of my body so that it could meet an ambitious goal. So are you.

You are a hero simply because you are making it through every day in the difficult circumstances you have been handed. You are also a hero because doing serious healing work deeply affects everyone around you. When you do the work necessary to live a healthy life, it inspires and moves every friend, relative, and health-care provider in your orbit in powerful and unpredictable ways.

In the airbrushed, Photoshopped world we live in, we are made to feel like losers and helpless victims for having any sort of frailty. That makes it hard to remember that you are a hero. I know that you are. Do whatever you can to remember it as well.

>>> *For Today* <<<
How does it feel to try on this identity as a hero? Hold in your heart for a few minutes today the knowledge that, whatever you think, I know that you are a hero who is fighting a tough battle every day. I'm with you 100 percent of the way.

X

Day 63
Talk About the Hardest Thing

Some people believe holding on and hanging in there are signs of great strength. However, there are times when it takes much more strength to know when to let go....

—Ann Landers

Sometimes being a hero may mean accepting a deeply painful reality and leading your loved ones to do the same. This book mainly addresses health goals like "I manage my MS so that I am symptom-free," "I am cancer-free and energetic," or "I can fully use my knee again." However, as we come to a close of this exploration of believing in both the wonder of now and the possibility of the future, the final health challenge that all of us will face rears its head: death. Even though it can be deeply upsetting to contemplate, an exploration of how to have confidence when handling serious health challenges would be incomplete without including what that might mean even in the face of death.

As the National Institutes of Health includes in an article on end-of-life issues, "Few of us are comfortable talking about death, whether our own or a loved one's. It is a scary, even taboo, subject for many.... This is normal—but death is normal, too. All of us will face it at some point."[18] It is because of both that taboo and the reality that we will all have to face it in one form or another that I want to address death here.

I want to share with you this potentially transformative idea: Although death is a wrenching reality that we fight against with our every fiber, if someday it comes time to accept it, and one has the time and presence of mind to do so, there are those who choose to approach it in the same way they approached life. They choose to approach it with the same five practices described in this book.

Take Charge

What would taking charge look like when facing death? It could mean working with your loved ones to gather all the information possible about your options and what to expect. It could mean advocating for yourself with healthcare providers and being clear about your preferences. It is even possible to create a health goal for death. It might sound something like "I will face death surrounded by loved ones, free of debilitating pain, and clear of mind for as long as possible so that I can say goodbye, connect with those I care about, and fully experience this last journey." That is a truly ambitious goal, which takes a great deal of commitment, confidence, and connection to even partially achieve.

Nurture Your Heart

At the end of life, if people have presence of mind, they often wind up in the position of being strong for everyone around them. That can be very isolating and make a terrifying experience even more challenging. In order to think clearly and stay connected to your loved ones, it is critical to have people with whom you can cry as long as you need, share your worries and fears, and explore options without having to take care of their feelings. Someone who has been taught how to do the listening partnerships described in Practice 2, Nurture Your Heart, would be particularly able to play that role.

»»» *For Today* ««<

Though discussing death and carrying out meaningful end-of-life rituals were part of traditional cultures for millennia, our modern society tends to avoid the issue until it's too late. Just thinking and speaking about death better equips us to handle it when the time comes for us or a loved one. Two good places to start are *Being Mortal* by Dr. Atul Gawande or *The Conversation* by Dr. Angelo E. Volandes. These two books thoughtfully explore how end-of-life issues are handled in the medical system today.

><

Day 64
Believing at the End of Life

One who wants to work on himself...needs to agree to stand from now for the rest of his life on this foundation of learning from all things, right up to his last day. He doesn't just die, rather he learns how to die.

—Rabbi Shlomo Wolbe

Believe

Even if you reach the heartbreaking point where you can no longer realistically believe in your ability to live past a certain time, there are still many things that you can choose to believe in. Like all things, it is possible to take a more-or-less optimistic approach to death. You get to decide. You could strive to believe that your family will be all right after you go; that you will stay closely connected to loved ones as you go; that you did what you were meant to do this time around on earth; and that, as painful as it is, it might be okay to let go. These are extremely difficult ideas to hold onto, but aiming to do so has given countless people comfort in their last days.

When facing death, many people also find great comfort in exploring reports of an afterlife and choosing to believe that they will be transitioning into some new experience rather than simply ceasing to exist. Nobody knows where truth lies in that realm. It can, however, provide enormous comfort in the darkest hours. Helen Keller clearly embraced this perspective when she said, "Death is no more than passing from one room into another. But there's a difference for me, you know. Because in that other room I shall be able to see."

Connect

Get all the support for you and your family that you can. Not everybody has the emotional capacity to be present with someone who is dying, but many people that stay away may do so because they don't want to get in the way or don't know how to help. If there are people that you want to be involved in helping out with food, childcare, logistics, or visits, be sure that somebody tells them that. They may think they are doing you a favor by giving you space.

Create Order

It may sound trivial to talk about legal documents in the context of death, but anyone who has experienced the death of a loved one with important documents missing or important issues unresolved will tell you that it can add enormously to the suffering of those left behind and even to the stress of the one who is dying. Taking the time to ensure that all the relevant legal documents are in place and all important decisions are addressed will give everybody more peace of mind to focus on what's really important.

Some of the documents to consider include a will, an advanced medical directive that specifies what medical actions should be taken if you are no longer able to make decisions for yourself, a healthcare proxy that authorizes a loved one to make decisions on your behalf if you are incapacitated, and a list of all your financial accounts, with their passwords and usernames. If you have children, planning ahead would also include leaving messages for them as well as clear guidelines for their care after you are gone.

I know that it can be scary to think about death. I debated whether to include this topic in a book focused on embracing life. I decided to in the hope that it helps us all to explore the idea that "Death is not the opposite of life, but a part of it"[19]—and equips us a little better to handle it when the time comes, ideally in the distant future, for us or a loved one.

>»» *For Today* ««<

Even if you are the picture of health, it is always a good idea to make sure that you have things in order in case of a crisis. Take a moment to think about the legal documents listed in today's entry. Do you have them all in order? If something happened to you today, would your family have the information they need? If not, take one step toward rectifying that.

)(

Day 65
Kris Carr's Story: Accepting Fear and Embracing Joy

I learned that courage was not the absence of fear, but the triumph over it.

—Nelson Mandela

In recent days we've talked about heroes and about death. Now I want to introduce you to one of my healing heroes, who has both faced death and seized life, Kris Carr. Kris is the founder of the Crazy Sexy Wellness Revolution. When she put the words *crazy*, *sexy*, and *cancer* together in the titles of her first book and movie, she bravely embraced the dichotomies that deep healing work often requires.

Kris embodies harnessing fear while celebrating joy; accepting the current health reality while working toward a healthier future; and loving what is, while working toward change. These are difficult, opposing realities to hold, but they're potent catalysts for emotional and physical healing.

In the winter of 2003, Kris was 31 and working in New York City when she developed strange aches and shortness of breath. By Valentine's Day, she was diagnosed with an inoperable stage 4 cancer called *epithelioid hemangioendothelioma*, a sarcoma that speckled her lungs and liver with tumors and lesions. There was and still is no standard treatment, but there has been limited reported success with surgery, chemotherapy, or radiation. Her doctors told her that she had about 10 years to live.

After her diagnosis, Kris acknowledges that one side of her was simply terrified by the doctors' prognosis. But, as she put it in a 2013 Super Soul Sunday interview on the Oprah Winfrey Network, "Then there was a side of myself; the fighting side of myself, the loving side of myself; that decided to reject that information and to get busy living...."[20]

Kris immediately got busy researching, visiting doctors and alternative healers, putting together a team, and crafting a healing path for herself. In consultation with her oncologists, she decided to forego treatments like chemotherapy and radiation, which had shown only limited success in treating her type of cancer. She took on a plant-based diet featuring whole foods and supplemented by lots of vegetable juices. She also incorporated regular exercise into her life, and made a decision to embrace joy and live her passions. In the 12 years since her diagnosis, she has published best-selling books, married the love of her life, renovated a small farm, and founded a wellness movement that has helped hundreds of thousands of people around the world to live healthier, more joy-filled lives.

Kris still has cancer and it is still incurable. How does she deal with fears about the future? As she explained in that same Super Soul Sunday interview, "I'm not a big believer in fearlessness, because fear is the thing that will get us to the doctor when we find a lump and fear has purpose. So fear is just a part of normal life. How can you use it? How can you go through it? How can you face it, surf it, ride it and then get to the other side of it? There are a lot of things that I am still afraid about. Cancer isn't really one of them. Even the thought of dying early and not being able to fulfill the rest of my dreams...doesn't scare me. What scares me is not trying."[21]

Kris remembers going to an annual checkup a few years back: "I felt tired in my bones. I felt like giving up. But, it wasn't giving up on my life, or my love, or myself, or my future. It was giving up this feeling of 'Until they say I am perfectly healthy, I am broken.' I looked around and decided that was a dragon that I would be chasing my entire life if I didn't change my thinking, because I may never be healthy on paper, but I am well."[22]

Kris continues: "[In 2013], I went to my 10-year check-up and I went in pretty anxious and got some pretty shocking news. I found out that my tumors had started to shrink and I was just so joyful. I had released my need to be in remission—for my own mental well-being. I had worked on truly loving what is, all parts of myself, whether there were tumors or not. Life is a terminal condition. We're all going to die. But, how many of us will truly live?"[23]

>>> *For Today* <<<
Take some time to learn more about Kris's journey and her healing philosophy at *www.kriscarr.com*.

><

Connect

When a person is singing and cannot lift his
voice, and another comes and sings with him—
another who can lift his voice—the first will be
able to lift his voice too. That is the secret of the
bond between spirits.

—Martin Buber

Now that you've worked on taking charge and believing in your dreams, it's time to get help to make them come true. The focus of this practice, Connect, is on how getting support can revolutionize your healing process. It's called *Connect* instead of *Get Support* because what is even more important than having meals delivered or your dishes done, is the heart connection that comes from bringing loved ones into your healing work and authentically sharing your challenges and victories with them. Dealing with a serious health condition can be one of life's most physically and emotionally isolating experiences. This sense of connection can give you confidence and lift you up in ways that nothing else can.

We all approach this topic from different perspectives and with different habits. Some of us are fiercely independent to a fault, and may be loathe to ask for or accept help of any kind. Others might have a bit of learned helplessness and are more inclined to give up or ask somebody else to do something for them as soon as the going gets tough.

Wherever you are on that continuum, the goal of this practice is not to get others to do things for you (except maybe some food preparation and a few loads of laundry—that would be nice). The goal is to get help so that you can do what you need to do for yourself: Put your healing work first and get your health back.

Day 66
Deepen Your Relationships to Deepen Your Healing

The study also offers a lesson for friends of people who have cancer, showing that small offers of help—like driving a patient to the doctor or offering to care for their children— can make a meaningful difference in the patient's survival.

—Tara Parker Pope, *New York Times*

I know that it's often not easy or comfortable to ask for help. But reaching out to your friends and family to bring them along on this ride can make an enormous difference in your healing.

› An analysis of 81 medical studies found that higher levels of social support had a positive impact on cardiovascular health, endocrine functioning, and immune systems.[1]

› Research has shown that elderly patients who had higher levels of emotional support had longer survival rates after a heart attack.[2]

› A study showed that married cancer patients were 20 percent less likely to die of their disease than single cancer patients; not just because they were married, but because of the extra social support they got from their marriage.[3]

The message is this: Having more people in your life who care about your health, are paying attention to it, and are supporting you to take care of yourself can vastly improve your health and, in some cases, save your life. These people do not need to be a spouse. They can be friends or family members. Ideally, you will have more than one. The key is to be willing to invite them in, to tell them about your struggles, your fears, your appointments, and your plans, so that they can help. It can be hard to make yourself vulnerable that way and some people may not respond the way that you would like. But it is the only route to having the kind of connections that will make a difference in your healing and, truly, in the rest of your life.

I was lucky. In addition to David, my husband, and a few friends, my older brother was right there with me all through my illness. He had successfully used diet to treat his own chronic illness, similar to mine. Even when it annoyed me, my brother regularly reminded me that when I was ready, an intense detoxifying diet might make a real difference to my health.

Finally, after years of conventional and alternative treatments that provided no relief, it was my brother's insistence that led me to explore the healing diet that ultimately brought me back to full health. I am forever grateful to him. Without our close relationship, I don't know if I would have been open to that healing approach, if I would have made the difficult lifestyle changes I needed to, or if I ever would have gotten well at all.

»» *For Today* ««

As you embark on this journey of increasing and strengthening your connections, take a few minutes to think about the people who you might want to invite along with you (or invite to get more involved than they already are). Think about how much you care for them and what you would do to help them improve their health if the tables were turned.

><

Day 67
Be a Leader—Ask for Help

Example is leadership.

—Albert Schweitzer

In our individualistic society, where the highest compliment is being called "self-made," we often regard accepting help as a sign of weakness. It follows that most of us have a hard time asking for help. Here is an interesting question: What single person in the world gets the most help to achieve his or her goals? I am pretty sure that would be someone like the president of the United States. The president has people who drive, shop, cook, clean, schedule, think, write, and even talk for him. Think about it. Having a wide variety of support to achieve important goals is not a sign of weakness. It's a sign of strength—of leadership.

Anyone who is trying to heal from a significant health challenge is pursuing an important goal as well, one deserving of a team just like the president has (well, maybe not quite as big). The goal of overcoming a health challenge is important simply because every person is important, is precious, and deserves to live to his or her full potential. Jewish tradition holds that every person is made *b'tzelem elokim*—that's Hebrew for "in the image of God." As far as I know, all major religions share this perspective that every individual carries a spark of the Divine in them—that all of our gifts and love are manifestations of the Creator's gifts and love.

When one person helps another achieve his or her health goals, they help to ensure that person's divine gifts are manifested in the world. If that's not important, I don't know what is.

On a more basic level, when a person is healthier, she can share her caring and skills with her friends, family, and broader community more easily, which benefits them as well. So as you work on your healing, keep in mind that you are working toward a goal that is important, not only to you, but—on many levels—to everyone around you. You deserve a team for that.

Building that team is not a sign of weakness or a burden on your friends and family. It is an act of visionary leadership. Any time you stand up and try to change your life for the better, you serve as an inspiring model for others. I am humbled by the changes that many people close to me have made in their lives as a result of seeing my healing process firsthand. From radically changing their diets, to taking more control of their children's healthcare, to successfully using physical therapy instead of surgery to address an old injury, many people have told me that my experience of committing to full health emboldened them to do the same.

>»> *For Today* «««

Imagine yourself leading your friends and family to a healthier and more connected future for all of you. What would that look like? Visualize it in as much detail as you can.

)(

Day 68
Do You Really Need Help to Heal?

Alone we can do so little. Together, we can do so much.

—Helen Keller

We have established that you and the president of the United States both deserve a team to meet your important goals. Now, let's clarify why you need that help to achieve your goal in the first place. In most cases, dealing with a significant health condition is a major organizational project that can require high-level skills like:

> Handling tough emotions (your own and others').

> Managing complicated data.

> Conducting in-depth research on treatment options.

> Setting up detailed schedules.

> Learning new food-preparation techniques.

> Negotiating a complex healthcare system.

> Managing complicated finances.

> Developing and maintaining a new exercise regimen.

> Communicating on sensitive topics with health professionals, friends, and family.

Plus, this may be a job that you have to do while you are sick—and guess what? There are no sick days. A corporation would assign a project of this size to a team of people. We all need and deserve the same. More focused health goals, like healing a nagging sports injury or losing 15 pounds, might not be as all-consuming, but they also become more achievable when you reach out for support.

Dr. Danielle Ofri, a professor at New York University and practicing physician, highlighted the problem in a *New York Times* article by listing the many tasks necessary for a 67-year-old patient with diabetes, hypertension, and high cholesterol to take care of his health:[4]

> Get five prescriptions filled regularly, including managing any hassles with the pharmacy or health insurance company.

> Make dietary changes to decrease salt and fat.

> Exercise three or four times per week.

> Schedule and attend frequent medical appointments.

> Check blood sugar regularly.

> Remember to take several pills every morning and evening.

That is no small feat. In fact, it is a series of major efforts every day and can only go better if more people are involved in a supportive way. No matter what your health goals are, your efforts to achieve them will be strengthened when you recruit more people to your team. Nobody should have to do this alone.

>»> *For Today* «««

Make a list of all the things that you would like to be doing on a regular basis to take care of your health better and achieve your health goal. Notice for a few minutes how much easier it would be to do those things with a team (or a bigger team than you already have) behind you.

)(

Day 69
Notice That You Are Not Alone

If you want to end your isolation, you must be honest about what you want at a core level and decide to go after it.

—Martha Beck

In addition to helping you get all the work of healing done, a support team serves as a reminder that you are not alone, and that you are valued and loved. Although it is an enormous help to have someone do your laundry and cooking or go to doctors' visits with you, the messages that your psyche gets from that support are equally important.

Anxiety, fear, depression, and self-doubt are frequent fellow travelers with serious health conditions. Those feelings can both suppress your immune system and mess with your head. They make it difficult to take the initiative necessary to move your healing forward. Having people committed to your healing and involved on a regular basis can be an important protection against some of the hard feelings that can derail you.

It is also good to notice that you are not alone, because, well, you aren't. You are doing your healing work in the context of myriad relationships with family, friends, colleagues, health-care providers, neighbors, and more. Each one of those relationships impacts your ability to heal in ways great and small. A family member can completely change to a no-sugar, no-salt diet to support your healing efforts, or insist on having a house stocked with chips and cookies, or anything in between. One friend may ask about your healing work regularly, bring meals occasionally, and offer to go to doctors' appointments. The sad reality is that one or two friends might disappear for a while because they find your health challenge too hard to handle.

One of the most moving examples I have seen of the way loved ones can impact our health is the many pairs of relatives and friends I have met at healing retreat centers. At the Hippocrates Health Institute in West Palm Beach, Florida, I met a 55-year-old woman who brought her frail and failing 90-year-old father and his 78-year-old wife all the way from Canada for three weeks to see how he might benefit from the plant-based diet and immune-boosting practices offered there. When he arrived, he was confined to a wheelchair and was not alert enough to fully converse with other guests. By the third week, with his daughter's constant attention, he was walking with a walker and engaging in banter with guests at every meal. It was remarkable to see what his daughter's commitment had done for his health. She was as happy as he was. "It's been challenging. But, I haven't gotten to spend this much time with him in decades. I feel like I'm in the process of getting my dad back," she said.

At the Kripalu Center for Yoga and Health in Stockbridge, Massachusetts, I met two women who had been friends for decades. One had a digestive disorder and had invited the other to join her for a three-day trip to begin a new yoga and nutrition program that she hoped would help address her symptoms. Every time I saw the two women at meals they looked so happy: laughing and talking excitedly. At our last meal there together, they told me that it was the first time they had had extended time alone together since they were both married almost two decades before. They were rediscovering their friendship as they learned new yoga stretches and recipes.

The common factor in both of those stories is that someone took the initiative and invited the other to join them in an effort to get healthy. The woman at Hippocrates invited her father and his wife to address his health, whereas the woman at Kripalu invited her friend to keep her company as she tried something new to address her own health.

There are people in your life who care about you and would like to be involved somehow in your healing. Don't wait for them. Invite them to join you. It doesn't need to be an invitation to a health retreat. It could be an invitation to cook healthy food together, help you think about your treatment options, or join a gym together.

Your choices impact your family, friends, and coworkers' choices. You may not be able to control them, but you do have significant influence. This is where leadership comes in. The more that you share thoughtfully with them about your healing work and invite them in, the more they will choose to join you in ways that will ultimately lead both you and them to a healthier and more connected future.

>»> *For Today* «<«
Take some time to think about whom you might invite to get more involved in your healing journey.

)(

Day 70
Get Out of Your Way

Be brave enough to accept the help of others.

—Melba Colgrove

For a long time, I resisted asking for or accepting help. I thought I was just too self-sufficient and strong to really need help. In hindsight, I see my underlying fear that if I was the one being supported, instead of the one supporting others, those others might not love or respect me as much.

Even though I am a pretty self-confident person, I just hadn't learned to value or love myself enough to make those tough asks. Like most people, I had been hurt enough in my life that when my armor of accomplishments and productivity were stripped away by illness, when I was stuck at home for hours a day, unable to work and barely able to raise my children, I felt a lot less confident about my inherent value. That made it hard to ask for help. I let fear stop me.

As I began to see things differently, I also came to see the messages I had gotten from my family that influenced me. My parents and my maternal grandmother, who lived with us, were all fiercely independent people. They were also all (my mother in particular, and to this day) extremely generous to others. Yet, like most people in our society, they tried to avoid receiving help themselves. We got the message that it was definitely way better to give than to receive, and that matters of health and family relationships were private.

I know that they meant well. They wanted to instill in their children a sense of independence and self-sufficiency, combined with a responsibility for caring for others, which they did. The only problem was that it also contributed to my difficulty in sharing my struggles and asking for help when I needed it. I don't mean to blame them for my challenges. I take full responsibility for my own decisions, as we all must. We will also all make better decisions if we take time to uncover our ingrained beliefs about receiving help and whether they still serve us.

Here are some examples of how I got in my own way and did *not* allow others to give me support in the early years of my illness: I did not accept the offers of neighbors to do regular food shopping for me. For a long time, I did not accept the generous offers of my parents and parents-in-law to pay for extra childcare when my sons were toddlers. I did not ask people to accompany me to healthcare providers' offices, even though I had read several times that it was a good idea. I did not let people cook for my family on a regular basis because it felt like too much to organize and too much to ask. I did not ask people to review treatment options with me because I didn't want to bother them.

I spent hours and hours alone, exhausted, scared, and confused, searching the Internet for a cure, going to a gazillion providers' offices looking for a diagnosis, and working with my husband to hold our family together without enough help and support—all because I couldn't ask for it. Doing it all by myself just made me sicker. That was a big mistake.

After I worked through my resistance, I began changing my behavior. I explained my health challenge to more people, accepted more help, and made it easier for friends and family to support me. That in turn enabled me to do the hard work of healing myself.

>»> *For Today* «<«
Are you asking for help where you can? Are there generous offers of help that you have turned down? Begin to explore why you've made those choices.

)(

Day 71
Jump In: What's Getting in the Way of Getting Connected?

A flood was approaching a man's village, but when a neighbor came to walk him to safety, he refused, saying, "God will save me." He refused again as the flood came closer and a wagon came to fetch him, repeating, "God will save me." The waters rose and a boat floated by, but the man refused a ride, saying again, "God will save me." As he sat on his roof with the waters about to engulf his house, he cried out to God, "Why have you abandoned me?" A voice from heaven replied, "I sent a neighbor, a wagon, and a boat. What else do you want me to do?"

—Unknown

Use this exercise to explore your feelings about getting more support. Take a few minutes to write whatever comes to your mind first for each prompt.

1. When I think about asking for support for my healing work, I feel....

2. When I think about asking for support with my healing, I think....

3. Attitudes toward receiving help in my childhood family were....

4. Other experiences I had receiving help or watching others receive help include....

5. Those experiences or attitudes may serve me in these way....

6. Those experiences or attitudes may limit me in these ways....

7. Going forward, I want to commit to changing how I think about getting help in this way....

)(

Day 72
See the Support Around You

You (Creator) open your hand and satisfy the desire of every living thing.

—Psalm 145

Imagine how different your life would be if you had someone helping you buy and prepare your food, joining you in an exercise regime, listening to you vent regularly about the challenges of getting healthy, reviewing treatment options, doing some dishes and laundry, and going to major doctors' appointments with you.

What feelings does that bring up for you? You might notice some feelings of isolation as you realize how alone you may have felt in your efforts to heal with whatever level of help you have now. You might also look at that list and think, "I could never do that. I could never ask for that kind of help." I understand that fear, but it's just not true. People, organizations, and groups are out there waiting to support you. Help is probably around if you look for it.

In today's quote, Psalm 145 says of God, "You open your hand and satisfy the desires of every living thing." I confess that the first time I read that I thought, "What a bunch of garbage." It is clear that every living thing's desires are not satisfied—not even close. Since then, with the help of some wise teachers, I have come to interpret that phrase differently. I believe that a beneficent force in the world (known to some as God) did set up the universe so that all the resources necessary to meet every real need do exist. I also believe that humans are partners in completing that creation. If we could all work together as effectively as possible, we do have the capacity to figure out how to use and distribute all the world's resources to meet everybody's needs. The human family is still working on figuring that out. We're just not there yet.

In our own lives, we can embrace the idea that every type of resource that we need to live a healing and healthy life is out there and available to us. That means that it is possible for us to find the support necessary to take care of ourselves and our family. Granted, it will take some work. It is also true that some people have easier access to those resources than others or have a greater need for assistance than others. But the resources we need are there for the taking for all of us.

With creativity, courage, and persistence, you can uncover resources and support that you never imagined. You have family members and friends who want to help, but don't know how, or don't know you need help. There is probably someone on your block; at your church, temple, or mosque; or in your workplace who would help if he or she knew you were in need. It's all out there for you if you are willing to take the initiative to get it (even if you may need help just to look for the help).

I want to give a shout-out to all those people and organizations providing fabulous support through cooking and exercise classes, online forums, support groups, government aid, meet-ups, and so much more. Get online, visit local health-food stores, and ask your healthcare providers for recommendations so that you can explore the landscape and see what's available. Joining groups, taking classes, or sharing information online, can give you the critical information, skills, emotional support, or logistical assistance that you need to achieve your health goals. Take advantage of what's out there.

»» For Today ««

Take a few minutes to repeat this phrase to yourself: *You open your hand and satisfy the desire of every living thing* or another similar phrase, if that is more comfortable for you. Notice any disbelief or discomfort that arises and let it go to the best of your ability. The more that you can believe that the resources you need to heal are out there, the more likely it is that you will find them.

)(

Day 73
Choose a Primary Support Person

"No—" said Harry quickly; he hadn't counted on this, he had meant them to understand that he was undertaking the most dangerous journey alone.

"You said it once before," said Hermione quickly, "that there was time to turn back if we wanted to. We've had time, haven't we? We're with you whatever happens."

—J.K. Rowling

For the next few days, we will explore several different ways that people can get involved in your healing work. Then, you can begin to choose which would be most helpful to you. Today, let's look at the role of a primary support person.

A primary support person is usually a close friend, life partner, parent, or adult child with whom you live or spend a lot of time. Ideally, he or she chooses to invest deeply in your health goal and join you on your journey as your copilot, helping you gather information, make decisions, and manage tough emotions. He or she can attend significant medical appointments with you and takes time with you to review treatment options and how to put them in place.

Early on in my illness, my husband, David, heard a famous story about Rabbi Aryeh Kaplan, who was known as Reb Aryeh, the *Tzadik* (Righteous One) of Jerusalem in the first half of the 20th century. Reb Aryeh and his wife went to the doctor together. When asked why they were there, Reb Aryeh pointed to his wife's leg and said, "Our knee hurts." David strove to make that idea the organizing principle for how he dealt with my illness. It wasn't just my illness and my problem to solve. It was something we were going through together, with me as the clear leader. I had felt terrible for all the suffering my illness was putting our family through. When David began to call it *"our* illness" or *"the* illness" instead of *"your* illness," it helped me feel less guilty, less alone, and more able to face what I had to do.

It took David a few years to fully internalize the "our illness" idea, but ultimately it was what made him a wonderful primary support person. He eventually joined me at doctors' appointments, agreed to dip into savings for my treatment, and helped shift our whole family to a healthier diet closer to mine. These pivotal changes were crucial in enabling me to take on the big changes I needed to make.

Here are some other ways that David and other exceptional primary support people assist their loved ones in taking charge of their health. They:

1. Strive to accept the seriousness of your health challenge, the extent to which it has limited your life or may do so in the future, and the fact that it is not your fault that you are struggling with it.

2. Commit fully to supporting your healing by following your leadership and making your health a top priority in your relationship with him or her for a number of weeks, months, or years, depending on your health challenge.

3. Avoid criticizing your choices or making you feel bad about your health, abilities, or choices in any way. I can't overstate this enough. People with serious health conditions are made to feel badly enough about themselves due to society's unhealthy messages about bodies and disabilities. Ideally, your primary support person is an antidote for those messages, not an echo.

4. Occasionally ask probing questions in a nonjudgmental, loving manner, to help you make the best decisions.

5. Support your difficult choices by taking on whatever elements of your healing lifestyle are possible, to make it easier for you to stick to them. (That may mean keeping the ice cream and pizza out of the house.)

If you are a single adult, or even if you have a life partner or other family member involved, it is often useful to have two or three people share this role, to avoid burnout. For example, one person can provide logistical support like helping with errands and meal preparation, as another offers primarily emotional support, and a third focuses on helping out with research and doctors' visits.

Keep in mind, if you have had a significant health challenge for a long time, it has likely been a big challenge for your primary support person as well. In addition to getting help for yourself, it is also important to help your primary support person get the emotional and logistical support he or she needs. You know that earlier point about your primary support person not criticizing you? He or she will likely be less cranky and critical if you have arranged for some meals to be cooked for you both and a neighbor's teenager to do the laundry and grocery shopping once a week.

Before we leave this topic, I want to acknowledge two things. First, most people do not automatically have a primary support person who is involved with their health condition in the way I have described here. Unless it's a life-threating situation, people often go to medical appointments, conduct research on treatments, and manage the logistics of their treatment alone. This is particularly true for people with chronic conditions. However, just because that is the way it usually is, doesn't mean that is the way it has to be. We are aiming for something different here. We are striving for a more connected and less isolated experience that enables you to transform your health, your relationships, and the lives of those around you.

Second, it may be that the person whom you would like to be your primary support person is not up to the task. It can be deeply upsetting when a loved one, such as a life partner or an adult child, is not able to support you in the way that you want. There are many different reasons this can happen. He or she might be in denial about the seriousness of your situation. He or she might not have the communication skills for the job or be uncomfortable in the role of caretaker. Maybe your relationship with him or her is strained for other reasons and can't handle the extra stress.

If you are experiencing this and would like him or her to get more involved in your healing work, you can discuss today's entry with him or her and see if there are any shifts with time. You can also share a powerful essay entitled "To the Partners," written by my husband, David. It's a letter of support and encouragement, combined with some gentle butt-kicking, to the partners of people with significant health conditions. It is a testimonial both to how difficult this can be for partners and to what a difference they can make. You can download "To the Partners" for free at *www.EverydayHealingforYou.com/tools.*

If, after all your best efforts, your loved one still isn't able to participate in the way you would like him or her to, do the best you can to accept it and, most importantly, don't blame yourself. Something is getting in his or her way. It's not your fault. Look to other friends and family members to provide the support you had hoped to get from him or her.

»»» *For Today* ««

Think about who your primary support person is or could be. Schedule a time to sit down with him or her, to share this piece, and to discuss how you can work together to move your healing forward. If there is not one obvious person, explore how you might get two or three people to share this role. Lastly, think about what emotional or logistical support your primary support person needs in order to participate fully in your healing work.

)(

Day 74
Hold Hands When You Head Into the Health-Care System

*Nobody should try to navigate the system alone.
Everyone should have what I call a health buddy who
goes along for routine checkups, annual tests and
who, during hospitalization, can serve as an extra
pair of eyes, ears, and perhaps hands. There's nothing
like having a friend or relative lending support,
encouraging you to tell the whole story, and helping
you make sense of what the doctor says. It doesn't take
a skilled person—just someone who can listen, absorb,
and care.*

—Dr. Marie Savard

Remember that book *All I Really Need to Know I Learned in Kindergarten*? It reminded us to "Hold hands when you cross the street." I second that, and would add: "Be extra sure to hold hands when you dive into the U.S. healthcare system." The maze of primary-care doctors, specialists, insurance snafus, prescription drugs, over-the-counter supplements, and alternative treatments is intense on the best of days and can be completely overwhelming on less-good days. In our individualistic society, we tend to soldier ahead into encounters with health providers largely on our own, reporting the results back to our loved ones after we return. As a general rule, only the oldest and youngest among us, or those facing possible life-or-death decisions, get much assistance and time from family members and friends to attend appointments and sift through complicated medical information. It doesn't need to be like that.

Inviting loved ones to go to healthcare appointments with you, help you research possible treatments, and think over options will create more allies who are invested in your path and your progress. The result will be better decisions, better health outcomes, and closer relationships.

Appointment Buddy

Although it is not always a common practice, it is vital that you have a friend or family member along at any health-provider appointment where you may be giving or receiving critical information. They can give you moral support, take notes, and help you remember which questions you wanted to ask. They will also have a much better understanding of your health challenge afterward and be able to support you more effectively in all your healing work.

Strategic Planning

There are big choices to be made on your path to health, like:

> Which treatment should I try?

> Which healthcare provider's advice should I take?

> Which nutrition plan is right for me?

> Is this program (or treatment) worth all this money?

> Can I possibly quit my job or cut back to half-time?

Don't make these decisions alone. You don't need someone else to do it for you, but you will be able to see your choices more clearly if you can talk over the options and vent your hopes and fears about them first with a good listener or two. They can listen to you work through tough feelings that may be clouding your thinking, as well as ask probing questions to help you think through different scenarios.

Research

The Internet is a curse and a blessing. The information there is invaluable, but its sheer volume is overwhelming. Assistance in sorting through the data on a particular health challenge, treatment, or lifestyle change is immensely helpful. Ask friends to come sit with you for an hour as you read and organize information. You may intend to sit down and do research on treatments every day, but you are much more likely to do it and do it productively, if you make an appointment with a friend to do it together.

>>> *For Today* <<<

Think about who you could invite to join your journey in these ways and how you might ask them.

)(

Day 75
Outsource the Details

Until we can receive with an open heart, we're never really giving with an open heart. When we attach judgment to receiving help, we knowingly or unknowingly attach judgment to giving help.

—Brené Brown

We've been looking at how friends and family can help you manage your healing work directly through going to doctors' appointments, doing research with you, and more. You could also use help with the other more mundane aspects of life.

Getting help to manage some of the work of running a home and feeding yourself can give you invaluable breathing room to get badly needed rest or to focus on your self-care practices. There are many ways that others can support you.

Errands

Some health challenges sap our energy and turn little things like grocery shopping or running errands into monumental efforts. In addition, some treatment or rehabilitation plans require setting up new systems, getting new equipment, learning whole new ways of eating, or relearning old skills. That takes an enormous amount of time and makes keeping up with all the details difficult.

Keep a list of errands that you haven't managed to do. That way you always have something to offer any friend who says, "How can I help?" You could also have one or two friends who come by once or twice per month to visit briefly and do a short errand for you. They could pick up items at the pharmacy, have copies made of your stacks of test results, or return an unwanted product you ordered online in the mail for you. Getting help with these details will reduce your stress, let you focus on your healing, and keep others in the loop about your healing efforts.

Housework

If someone could come do your laundry, dishes, and a little cleaning on a regular basis, you would have a lot more energy for the healing and self-care you need to do. If you have children and are debilitated at all by your health condition, having someone else deal with housework also allows you to use more of your limited time and energy to focus on your children.

There are several ways you can outsource housework. You could pay a responsible neighborhood tween to come help out a few hours per week. One or two people in your household might not be meeting their potential in the housework department. This is a good time to ask them to pick up their game. You could ask a couple of good friends if they could each come by to hang out with you and sort and fold laundry a couple times per month each. For a few years we had a student live with us in exchange for several hours of grocery shopping, laundry, dishes, and childcare each week. That had its pros and cons, and not everybody has the room to do it. It was, though, a lifesaver when we desperately needed it.

Meal Preparation

Having meals prepared for you can be a lifesaver, especially if you are physically weakened and need rest, or if you have to prepare a special diet for yourself and a whole other set of meals for your family. It is also important to delegate to one or two people the whole job of organizing people to take turns delivering meals. There are several Websites that make it easier (*www.lotsahelpinghands.com* and *www.mealtrain.com* are just two examples).

If you are on a special diet, have your organizers post suggested recipes and clear instructions on the Website for your food-preparers. You can also include directions about when and how to drop off meals that make it convenient for you. If you don't, you might spend almost as much time each day giving instructions to your helpers as you would making a meal.

Childcare

The young people in our lives are a blast. They are also exhausting. If you have children, get help taking care of them to enable you to do the self-care and get the rest you need. You may not want to give up precious time with your children or entrust them to somebody else, but this investment now in improving your health will be a gift that will only benefit your children in the long run.

Eldercare

If you are responsible for caring for an older family member, explore ways to take some of that stress off you as you focus on your healing. Perhaps other family members, friends, community members, or paid health aides can pick up the slack for you for a while. Don't sacrifice your health. There's always a better solution. It just might take some time and creativity to find it.

>>> *For Today* <<<

Call a friend to brainstorm about ways that you could set up some of this support for yourself.

><

Day 76
Healing Is Expensive—Ask for Help

American culture in particular has instilled in us the bizarre notion that to ask for help amounts to an admission of failure. But some of the most powerful, successful, admired people in the world seem, to me, to have something in common: they ask constantly, creatively, compassionately, and gracefully.

—Amanda Palmer

Money is a tricky topic. You might prefer to do a lot of really unpleasant things (drinking turpentine and sliding bamboo shoots under your nails come to mind) rather than ask people for money. But the reality is that the healthcare market is a pricey place. As you know, trying to heal can absolutely break the bank. If you are unable to work, or decide to cut back your work hours to facilitate your healing, you face these added costs with a reduced income. It's not a pretty picture. Here is a list of possible sources of financial support:

> › Government aid is there to help people who need it. If you think you might be eligible, community health centers, community service centers, local nonprofits, and local government offices have programs to help you navigate the system

to apply for government aid, including food aid, financial support, Social Security benefits for disabilities, subsidized health insurance, or affordable housing. Don't be shy if you might be eligible. You or your family have probably paid taxes that cover this aid for years. Now you need it, like millions of good people before you.

> Apply for financial aid for the tuition for any health-oriented program you attend.

> If you have any, let your more financially comfortable friends or relatives know that you need help. (Parents and grandparents are sometimes a good first choice.) If they have it, ask for it.

> Have a friend do a fundraiser in your name by sending out group e-mails or doing some crowdfunding online to help you out. Two Websites that help people crowdfund for medical conditions are *www.giveforward.com* and *www.gofundme.com*. Check them out to see the many things people are successfully getting support for.

> Cut out other costs in your budget to afford your health care. Your budget may already be bare bones and there is nothing left to cut. But if that is not the case, look for what can go. You (or some in your family) may not want to change your lifestyle, but if it might enable you to get back your full health or even save your life, I think everyone would agree that it's worth a year or two of staycations, dinners at home, and hand-me-down clothes. That might not cover all the additional costs, but it can help. You just need to make the case.

> It may make sense to dip into savings or retirement funds, if you are lucky enough to have any. I can't recommend that anyone do this because it is always a risk. However, in the long run, nothing is more important than your health. If you can't enjoy it or you family can't enjoy it with you, what is the point of all the cash?

It may feel easier to ask for money if you ask for the specific thing the money will be used for. Often, asking for funding to pay for one month's-worth of childcare or one month of housework and takeout food is more comfortable than asking for the same amount of money directly. I completely understand that asking for money is difficult. You can heal on a budget, but cash can be helpful, if you can get it.

>>> *For Today* <<<
If you need it, are there any sources of financial support that you haven't tapped yet, that you might be able to now? Brainstorm with friends and family about this question. If necessary, could you ask a friend to raise an appropriate amount of money for you through an event or an online crowdfunder? Which friend could you ask? If you do need that kind of help, but your first thought is "Are you crazy?" what gets in the way of asking or accepting that help? Would you do the same for your friend(s) if the tables were turned?

)(

Day 77
Find a Role Model

Find someone who has a life that you want and figure out how they got it. Read books. Pick your role models wisely. Find out what they did and do it.

—Lana Del Rey

One of the most essential, but overlooked, types of support you can get is finding successful role models—people who have or had a health condition similar to yours and have significantly improved their health the way that you want to improve yours.

Successful role models can save you years of struggle by helping you choose an effective healing path sooner. These people can be fountains of wisdom and support, and can help you think outside of your particular box and explore new modes of healing. They can introduce you to effective healing regimes or medical treatments, help you avoid reinventing the wheel, and give you valuable tips on adopting any new self-care practices or managing any treatment that you choose.

I want to acknowledge that doing the research necessary to find these people can take time and be emotionally draining, and that you will find more dead ends than helpful leads. Healthcare is not one-size-fits-all. What worked for someone else may not work for you. But, it might. And, after you've weighed any risks and checked in with your healthcare advisors, it may well be worth a try. It's a good idea to get someone to do the research with you occasionally, and to keep expectations low at the beginning of the search.

I wish that I had focused on finding these role models earlier in my quest for whole health. In late 2007, after five years of trying countless alternative and conventional treatments, I decided that I wasn't going to try another health intervention until I found at least two people with chronic Lyme disease and/or chronic fatigue syndrome who had been completely healed by it. Within a few months, I found a handful of people who had been completely cured by the healing lifestyle that I eventually adopted. Six months after I found and spoke with them, I was well on my way to full health. One of them was also a health coach. Doing a series of sessions with her was instrumental to me in successfully taking on my new diet and lifestyle. I simply could not have taken on that difficult change without their example, encouragement, and mentoring.

To make this research effective and to avoid scams and dead ends, you want to look—not just for treatments—but for individuals who meet very specific criteria and with whom you can talk, people who:

> Had or have your health condition or a set of symptoms similar to yours.

> Have fully achieved the health goal that you are trying to achieve.

> Have been in their new, improved healthier state for at least one full year, preferably two.

> Do not seem to be trying to get rich off of selling a "miracle cure." Respectfully marketing a book or offering coaching is great, but be wary of hard-sellers or people who refuse to give away their "secret" until you pay them a large amount.

> Are available to contact by e-mail or phone to set up a short conversation.

> Sound balanced, grounded, and trustworthy when speaking to them.

So, how does one go about looking for these healing models? The following is a list of possible routes to try, keeping in mind the two seemingly opposing truths that 1) There are a lot of scammers out there, and 2) You never know who or what might give you the information and inspiration you need, so keep an open mind.

> Do an Internet search of your health condition plus key words like *cured*, *healed*, *got off medications*, *symptom-free*, *pain-free*, *diet*, *exercise*, *treatment*, *my story*, or a specific treatment that you are interested in.

> Ask in chat forums, Facebook groups, and e-mail LISTSERVs on your health condition.

> Ask healthcare providers whom you trust for leads.

> Ask your friends and family to keep their eyes and ears open.

> Make it a high-priority research project. Think like an investigative journalist.

> Always keep a list of treatments you want to try and people whom you want to contact.

> When you find someone, run any new treatment they recommend past one or two healthcare providers whom you trust and who are also committed to keeping an open mind.

Of course, this search does not guarantee success. Yet, no matter what happens, you will discover some amazing, inspiring people and learn a great deal about the healing options out there for you. You may even find the key to unlock the best health you could possibly imagine. You don't have to do your healing work alone. You deserve mentors and role models to help you through it.

>>> *For Today* <<<

If you haven't recently, take one of the steps listed previously with an eye to finding not just a path to better health, but people who can vouch for that path and help you follow it.

><

Day 78
Getting Support to Recover From Cancer Treatment

When you ask for what you need and receive what people and the world have to give, you open up pathways you couldn't see before, stimulate your imagination in ways that could not happen before, and have energy that was not previously available to you.

—Amanda Owen

Now that we've gone over a bunch of different types of support, let's look at what a support system for a 46-year-old mother of two could look like to help her recover her strength and energy when, two years after cancer treatment for breast cancer, she is still plagued by debilitating fatigue and body aches that had started during her surgery and chemotherapy. When she decides to establish a less-stressful, healthier lifestyle and choose a new treatment plan to get her health back, she might put together a support team like this:

Primary Support Person

Her husband could agree to 1) live by whatever healing diet she chooses when he eats in the house, so as to limit the temptations she faces; 2) take their children to his parents' home over the summer for two weeks so that she can organize everything she needs for her new healing effort; and 3) significantly cut back on the family's expenses and lifestyle, and get a small loan, so that she could not work for at least one year.

Emotional Support

She could choose a few friends who were good listeners and train them in doing the listening partnerships described in Practice 2, Nurture Your Heart. If she scheduled at least one check-in phone call each day with one of these friends and one longer, in-person listening partnership each week, she could get help with managing her emotions so that they didn't manage her. Her friends would also have time to work through what was going on in their lives, so this emotional support would be mutually helpful and deepen those relationships significantly.

Appointment Buddies

Her husband could join her at significant medical appointments, and one or two close friends could serve as backups when her husband couldn't make an appointment.

Meals, Childcare, Housework, and Errands

A friend could set up a Web page on *www.lotsahelpinghands.com* to allow friends, family, and work colleagues to sign up online to bring food, help with shopping and dishes, run an errand, or pick up her children at school, even just a couple of times per week.

Strategic Planning

She could meet every few weeks or as needed with her husband or one of her close friends to go over her current treatment options, plans, and strategies.

>>> *For Today* <<<

What elements of this support plan could you incorporate into your own healing work?

)(

Day 79
Getting Support to Lose Weight

Gracious acceptance is an art—an art which most never bother to cultivate. We think that we have to learn how to give, but we forget about accepting things, which can be much harder than giving.... Accepting another person's gift is allowing him to express his feelings for you.

—Alexander McCall Smith

What about a 35-year-old man who weighs 275 pounds and is pre-diabetic? What support could he get to lose 100 pounds so he could feel better and ward off serious health problems in the future?

Emotional Support

If relevant to his needs, he could join Overeaters Anonymous (OA) to have a regular place to share ideas and experiences with people working through similar issues, and do daily phone check-ins with a friend, his OA sponsor, or with other OA participants.

Exercise Buddy

He could invite two friends to train together to walk/run a 10K charity race 12 months out, and walk/run with them three to four times per week for several months.

Meal Preparation

He could work with a friend to organize biweekly meetups where all the participants bring a family-sized serving of a healthy meal that meet his diet criteria, to be divided up into smaller portions so that each person goes home with a bunch of containers offering several healthy dinner options for the week.

Losing that much weight would still be challenging, but with this kind of support in place, he would have a much better shot at reaching his goal.

»»» For Today «««

What elements of this support plan could you adapt for your healing work?

)(

Day 80
Jump In: What Support Could You Use to Heal?

It always seems impossible until it's done.

—Nelson Mandela

Having looked at a couple of hypothetical support plans, you might be saying, "That's very nice, but there is no way I will ever get all that help from my friends and family. They have their own busy lives and their own challenges to handle." Maybe they don't even believe or realize that you are sick or in pain or dangerously overweight. Maybe you have recently moved and don't have a network of friends and family around you. (Thank God for phones, e-mail, social media, and Skype. Your old networks can still give you support.)

Or, you may be thinking that anyone who could organize that kind of support must have better organized, richer, or more generous friends than you have. Happily, that is not true.

The secret ingredient required to set up that kind of support is leadership. It takes bringing in people one-by-one to create a team to support you on your path to whole health. Remember, though: progress, not perfection. You don't need to do it all at once. If you use the ideas from this section on getting connected to engage just one friend or relative in your process, that will help you cut your isolation and move you forward toward more support and more breakthroughs in your healing work.

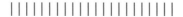

Step 1. Think about all of the different kinds of support you would like from your friends, family, and wider community in getting healthy. The sky is the limit. What might help you achieve your health goals?

Step 2. Make a list of all the things you imagine. Try to write as many as 20 different ways you could get help. Include support that is mutually beneficial like exercise buddies, meal meetups, or listening partnerships. You don't need to ask for all that right now or ever. Just notice how much support you could use. You may not get it all, but the more you notice what you could use, the more likely you are to ask, and the more likely you are to get the help you need.

Step 3. Address any lingering doubts you may have that it is okay to ask for help. Come up with at least one family member or friend who you think might be willing to get involved. Call him or her today just to talk about your health and brainstorm ways that you could take better care of yourself. You can share some of the ideas in this section, if that's helpful. If you're not comfortable asking for help, don't ask for anything yet. Just bring him or her in a bit more on your journey and see what happens.

✕

Day 81
Four Steps to Ask for What You Need

If you don't go after what you want, you'll never have it.
If you don't ask, the answer is always no. If you don't step
forward, you're always in the same place.

—Nora Roberts

Now that you have made your list of the support you could use, you may still be wondering, "How do I set all that up?" These things work differently for every person, but from my own and others' experience, I have found that following these four steps helps immensely in setting up effective support to move you forward in your healing. You don't need to use all four steps in every situation. Just being aware of them and using them when appropriate makes it easier to ask in the first place, and improves the quality of both the support itself and your relationship with the people whom you are asking.

Step 1: Inflation

Sometimes, you may need to inflate your own sense of personal worth and power in order to take leadership in this way. We all have some self-confidence issues and if you have been struggling for months or years with a health challenge, your self-worth might be a bit like a deflated inner tube. Pump it up!

Step 2: Explanation

Explain to your friends and family how limited you really are by your health challenge, or how limited you may be in the future if you don't address it now. Tell them in detail what your symptoms are like, how it limits your life, or how scared you are about the treatments and prognosis you are facing. Let them know what it is like for you to suffer in this way. This is not complaining. This is giving them information so that they can understand you better, help you, and have a closer relationship with you.

Step 3: Education

Educate them generally about your health challenge: what it is, what your treatment options are so far, and what different healing options you want to explore going forward. Giving them thorough information increases their confidence in their ability to help and also prevents them from asking lots of uninformed questions later that can, frankly, get pretty annoying.

Step 4: Invitation

After you lay the groundwork with the first three steps, thoughtfully invite them to get involved in your healing effort, to be part of this journey that can change all of your lives.

>>> *For Today* <<<
Review the long list of support you made yesterday and take some time to imagine how much further you could get in your healing work if you were able to put even a few of those elements into place.

)(

Day 82
Step 1. Inflation—Pump Up Your Self-Worth

We're miserable because we think that we are mere individuals, alone with our fears and flaws and resentment and mortality.

—Elizabeth Gilbert

I don't need to tell you that our modern society promotes some messed-up values. In the big-box, super-size, reality-TV world we live in, how much money you have is more important than how you behave. We value people based on their productivity, wealth, fame, and appearance, rather than their inherent preciousness as human beings. Your ego can take a real beating in that environment if your ability to work has been limited by illness or pain; if you feel like you are not looking your best; or if you are carrying some extra weight. Alternatively, if you don't feel that your ego has taken a beating, you may have internalized all of our society's messages about self-reliance enough to think that asking for help is a sign of weakness, when it really is the opposite. It is a sign of brave leadership.

Either way, you could probably use some pumping up before you ask people to join your support team. Build up your sense of self-worth and remind yourself how precious you are and how much you are loved.

There are many ways to accomplish this. Spending time with people who love you and treat you well is always a good one. Remembering times when you felt truly loved and valued or felt that way deeply about yourself is another. Use whatever spiritual or counseling practices you find meaningful to ensure that you are feeling as good about yourself as possible. See Day 83 for a few useful exercises to supplement that.

For Today

Think or write about what a good human being you are, how much you are loved, and how valuable you are just for being you. If you have some resistance here and don't feel so valuable or loved, write or talk about it with a friend, and set aside some time to use your best emotional and spiritual tools to work on remembering how precious you are.

>(

Day 83
Jump In: Inflation—Some Quick Reminders That You Are Worth It

People should be nice to you, Leonard. You're a human being. You should expect people to be nice.

—Matthew Quick

Step 1: Scan your memory and write three nice things that people have said to you or about you that really touched you. They can be as simple as the fact that you make your friend laugh or that your partner loves your smile.

Step 2: Scan your memory again and write down three memories in which you have felt particularly close to or appreciated by the people whom you were with in that memory.

Step 3: Scan your memory again and write down three successes that you have had of which you are very proud. They can be large or small, private or public, recent or long ago, and in any facet of life. It doesn't matter as long as they make you proud.

Step 4: Take some time to regularly meditate on, or just think about, any of these memories as often as you can. Relive the positive emotions they evoke and really feel how appreciated, loved, or confident they make you feel.

)(

Day 84
Step 2. Explanation—Don't Suffer Alone

If we have no peace, it is because we have forgotten that we belong to each other.

—Mother Teresa

I cannot tell you how many times I have heard (or said myself), "My friends just don't understand how sick I am." Or: "My family doesn't understand my illness at all. It's too painful for them to really face it." Or: "They think that if I just had more discipline, I could drop all this weight. It's not that easy!" The only way they will understand better is if you tell them, show them, or get someone else to tell them for you. Even then, some people will never really get it. But most of your family and friends can come a long way with some guidance.

This step and the next one (education), are particularly important if you have an invisible health challenge like chronic fatigue, fibromyalgia, severe allergies, multiple sclerosis, diabetes, chronic pain, or a sleep disorder. In those situations, because you don't look the way people expect a "sick" person to look, they often don't understand that your health is truly compromised. Friends and family may not understand that you need help or may not be sure how they can help. It's an extra burden on you and it shouldn't be that way. But it is. The only way they will understand is if you explain. They need your leadership.

In order to explain your health challenge, it is useful to come up with a vivid description to which the listener can relate. Here is the short explanation that I came up with to help people understand my symptoms when I sensed that they were skeptical that I was experiencing anything more debilitating than the sleep-deprived state of exhaustion thrust on most parents of young children:

Imagine how you would feel if you pulled two all-nighters in a row, staying up for work with only an hour or so of sleep. On the third day of almost no sleep, you would be achy, exhausted, cranky, and a bit spacey, right? You would probably be able to function if you had to, but everything would be a real effort and you would feel like you were just trying to survive the day. For the last six years, that's how I've felt on my good days. I am lucky enough to feel like that and be able to function about half the time. The rest of the time I feel like someone on the last day of the flu, when the fever is gone but the body aches, muscle weakness, and deep fatigue still take you out of the game. On those days, making a fist, washing my hair, or walking around the block are all big challenges.

That seemed to give people a fairly clear picture.

»»» For Today «««

What are the two things about your health condition that others have the hardest time understanding? How would you like to explain those things to family and friends to help them understand better?

><

Day 85
Jump In: Explanation—Tell Your Story

Stories are bridges from one mind to another.

—Martha Holloway

Because explaining your health challenge over and over again can get old, it's useful to write a page or two describing it, how it affects your life, and your physical and emotional experience of it. It can also be a very cathartic experience. Writing your story makes it more real, particularly if you have an "invisible illness." Describing it in writing makes it more concrete and helps you avoid those feelings of "being crazy" that are thrust on anybody with a long-term health condition.

Step 1. Write one to three pages to share with people close to you to help them understand your circumstances. You can include things like:

- How long you've had your condition.
- How your condition limits you.
- How it affects your daily life.
- Your fears.
- Your hopes.
- Your plans.

Step 2. Share your story with friends and family members to help them understand. It's best to arrange to talk with the person right after they read it, so that you don't feel left exposed with no reaction and so that they can ask questions. Often, when those who love us are not offering support or compassion, it is simply because they don't understand that we need it. Explain it to them.

><

Day 86
Step 3. Education—Share Information

Too often we underestimate the power of a touch, a smile, a kind word, a listening ear, an honest compliment, or the smallest act of caring, all of which have the potential to turn a life around.

—Leo Buscaglia

If you have had your health challenge for a while, the number of hours that you have sat in healthcare providers' offices, read up on various treatment options on the Internet, gone to support groups, tried various treatment plans, or just sat and thought about it all, should probably qualify you for at least a master's degree on the topic. You have a wealth of knowledge about your health challenge and how you might turn it around. If your diagnosis is a more recent event, you are still probably way ahead of your family and friends in educating yourself about it.

Sharing some of that information with your loved ones can empower them to get more involved in your healing effort. You don't need to organize it into a fancy presentation. Just take the time to jot down at least four things you would like your family and friends to know about your health condition, plus your ideas for the next steps on your path to whole health.

When I decided to bring in more people on my healing journey, I wanted them to understand how poorly understood my illness was, what some of the ideas were about what caused it, how low the cure rate was, how intense the side effects were for many of the treatments, and how I planned to move forward on choosing my next treatment plan. Showing them statistics and stories about chronic fatigue syndrome and chronic Lyme disease helped them understand the seriousness of the illness and that I really was sick, in spite of the fact that I "looked fine."

When our friends and family don't offer to help us in our healing, it often stems from feeling uninformed and helpless because they don't know what the options are. Arm them with information and make them feel a part of your team. It will go a long way toward getting them involved and make them more effective team members when they do join in.

>»> *For Today* «««
What are the four basic things about your health challenge
that you would like people on your support team to know?

)(

Day 87
Step 4. Invitation—Make the Ask

*When we were children, we used to think that when we were
grown-up we would no longer be vulnerable. But to grow up
is to accept vulnerability.... To be alive is to be vulnerable.*

—Madeleine L'Engle

It may not be easy to talk about the true dimensions of your health condition. It may not be easy to ask for help. In an ideal world, neither of these would be especially challenging. We would experience something difficult and simply ask for help, with no shame or guilt that we should be able to do it ourselves. But we don't live in that world yet.

Happily, once you've done the previous three steps (Inflation, Explanation, and Education) with whomever you are closest, the offers of help often come naturally and you can move easily into the next step of Invitation.

This step of expressly inviting people to join you in your healing work is essentially a matching game. You match people on your team with the support role you would like each of them to play. It is usually better to have a specific role in mind and ask for that outright than to throw it open and ask how someone would like to be involved. For example, your father might want to go with you to healthcare appointments, but that might not be your first preference. Or your friend whose cooking you don't love might offer to make meals. At the same time, if they have another idea of how they would be comfortable helping, be open to exploring that as well.

How do you figure out the best matches? You can go back to the list you made of types of support you would like, and write the name of a friend or family member who you think might be willing to help out with that type of support next to each one. Then, think about how and when you will do the inviting.

It is also important to be prepared for someone to say *no* and to give them the room to do so if they need to. You can always ask why and explore how else it might work for them to be involved in your healing. Asking with the open recognition that people might need to say *no* protects you from disappointment and them from feeling obligated.

If you do get a *no*, don't let that discourage you and prevent you from continuing on. Anybody who has gone through a serious health crisis will tell you that some people who they thought would really be there for them just failed to show up, whereas others who they hadn't expected to get involved at all were huge sources of support. Remember: The resources are out there. You just need to uncover them.

One great way to invite people to get involved that I have seen work many times is gathering a few close friends or family members together to plan what kind of support you need and where you might get it. When a friend of mine was facing a difficult cancer prognosis, I joined her, five other friends, and her husband to plan how to help them with childcare, meals, and financial support in the coming months.

Through brainstorming and activating all of our networks, in the next two weeks we supported them to find a wonderful part-time nanny, raise tens of thousands of dollars, set up daily rides to preschool for their sons, and arrange for dinners to be delivered indefinitely. They said that the logistical and financial help was wonderful, but even more transformative was the sense of being cared for by their communities during an extremely difficult time.

>>> *For Today* <<<
Choose one particular piece of support that you think will make a big difference to you. Decide who you are going to ask, how you are going to prepare for it (think about if and how you are going to do Inflation, Explanation, or Education first), exactly what you want to ask them, and when you are going to ask them. Or consider inviting two or three friends over to brainstorm about all this with you.

)(

Day 88
Gift Your Loved Ones With You

Fear defeats more people than any other one thing in the world.

—Ralph Waldo Emerson

As you consider inviting others to get involved in your healing work, some fears may be coming up—perhaps fears of embarrassing yourself, of seeming presumptuous, of being a burden, or of making people uncomfortable. That's normal. As I've already discussed, our society has led us to believe that asking for help is a weak, selfish thing to do, instead of the sign of leadership that it really can be.

Here's a new way to think of it: You are asking something of your friends and family, but you are also offering them four precious gifts.

> First, you are offering them the opportunity to deepen their relationship with you by joining in this effort as you make yourself vulnerable to them through sharing your hopes and concerns about your healing.

> Second, they will get to be part of an effort to radically change someone's life. People don't often make big changes in their lives beyond a new job, relationship, or location. To be intimately involved in another person's journey as they take charge of their life and steer it in a new direction is a priceless opportunity from which they will learn and grow immensely.

> Third, it's not a one-way street. Depending on what kind of support you need, getting involved in your healing work often directly benefits your friends and family. If you invite a friend who has been trying to set up a new exercise routine to join you at the gym twice per week, that's not imposing on her; that's offering her an opportunity. Even when your friends or family are not obviously benefiting from involvement as in that exercise-buddy example, they are still likely to learn a great deal through the experience. Whether they learn how to make a better salad, gain new insights into acceptance and perseverance, or discover how to run a medical appointment productively, they will grow from the experience along with you.

> Fourth, there are few things more meaningful than making a difference in the life of someone we love. These people have probably watched you struggle for months or even years with little sense of how to help. By giving your loved ones specific instructions of how they can support you, you are presenting them with a gift they have been waiting for. They don't have to sit by and feel helpless. They can do something! As long as you invite them with thoughtfulness and love, they will appreciate that you have offered them this opportunity.

>>> *For Today* <<<

Imagine that (God forbid) your life partner, child, parent, or close friend had the health challenge that you are facing now. Would you want them to read this book and think: *Too bad I can't ask anybody for more help?* Or would you want them to come to you with this chapter and say, "Can we talk?" Just as you care about them, they care about you and want to be involved, even if they don't know it yet. Come up with just one person who you can call, share some of this chapter with, and ask for help in brainstorming how you might set up more support for yourself.

)(

Day 89
Jump In: Map Your Healing Support Team

Teamwork is the secret that makes common people achieve uncommon results.

—Ifeanyi Enoch Onuoha

Create a chart like the following with four columns: the types of support you need, who you think would be good for that support, exactly what you want to ask them to do, and how you want to invite them. See the following headings for examples.

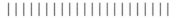

Type of Support	Who	Specifics	How to Invite
After-school childcare.	Beth—friend and parent at children's school.	Organize parents of your children's friends to each schedule one after-school playdate with your child(ren) once a month to get several afternoons covered.	Ask for a phone conversation or visit to explain, educate, and invite.

Type of Support	Who	Specifics	How to Invite
Exercise buddy.	Justin— close friend.	Meet you at the gym to work out two to three times per week.	Set a time to get together to explain, educate, and invite.
Accompaniment to health-provider visits.	Cheryl and Jennifer (close friends).	Go to two appointments each as you interview specialists to choose one for your next phase of treatment.	Ask if all three of you can get together for an hour or more, so that you can talk with them about your health condition and how they can help.

><

Day 90
Jump In: Notice Your Deep Connections

"Why did you do all this for me?"[Wilbur] asked. "I don't deserve it. I've never done anything for you."

"You have been my friend," replied Charlotte. "That in itself is a tremendous thing."

—E.B. White

Inviting people to get involved in your healing like this may seem daunting at first but, as I've said, once you have done the first three, the Invitation step often largely takes care of itself. You are feeling confident in your friend or family members' love, which brings their feelings of love for you to the fore. They are feeling connected to you by your willingness to show your real struggles and usually ask at some point, "What can I do to help?"

As we close this section on connecting, I will just ask again: If the tables were turned and a close friend or family member were healing from a health challenge, wouldn't you want him or her to ask you for help and give you clear instructions on how to do it? If you can't ask for help for you, do it for your loved ones. They are waiting for you.

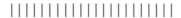

In case you still feel like you really don't want to or just can't ask friends or family for any significant support, try this:

Step 1: Imagine that, instead of you, it is a close friend who is having a hard time asking for and accepting as much help as he could use. Write a short letter to that friend to try to convince him to ask for and accept help. Tell him how loved, valuable, and precious he is; how much all of his friends and family want to help; and how much it will benefit him and all of them in the long run.

Step 2: Take the letter and replace the name of the person to whom you wrote it with your name. Now read the letter to yourself.

)(

Create Order

The world is not to be put in order. The world is order. It is for us to put ourselves in unison with this order.

—Henry Miller

In Practice 2, Nurture Your Heart, I shared the idea that having a hard time sticking to a self-care routine like daily exercise or healthy eating doesn't mean that you are inherently lazy or disorganized. It just means that some emotional or logistical blocks are getting in your way.

As a disorganized night owl with bad procrastination habits and more than a drop of anxiety, I had plenty of blocks of both kinds to overcome before I could commit to my healing path.

In this section, I want to share with you the wisdom that enabled me and many others to identify and overcome the logistical obstacles that got in our way of getting healthy. In the process, I hope that you will also see that creating order is about more than just getting organized. It's about recognizing and cherishing what is truly important: our health, our relationships, and our purpose on Earth.

Day 91
How Can Order Help You Heal?

> *Picture a pearl necklace with a small clasp. Which is more essential—the clasp or the pearls? At first glance the pearls are more essential. But, without the clasp all the pearls would scatter and all that would be left is the chain—thus the clasp seems more essential. A person is like a collection of pearls—he is full of potential, talents, character traits, and virtues. Seder [order] is similar to the clasp on the necklace. Without Seder all his virtues and talents scatter and he is left empty.*
>
> —Rabbi Simcha Zissel Ziv

Increasing order in your life unlocks potential. Without order, we can't make the best use of all of our skills and talents (or time, belongings, and money). Overcoming a major health challenge can require all the resources we have. Putting a little more order into your life makes it easier to tap those resources.

Having grown up fairly disorganized, with a flair for getting things done in a last-minute rush, I confess that I associated clear desks and neat homes with vacuous people who had nothing better to do than file papers and color-coordinate their sweater piles. I have now come to understand that neat desks and organized closets allow for more time and peace of mind to give attention to that which is most important, including taking care of one's health.

Marilyn Paul is the author of the best-selling *It's Hard to Make a Difference When You Can't Find Your Keys* and a brilliant leader on creating order in your home and work life. She helped me to see that being organized doesn't just mean looking good or being neat: It means managing your life well so that you can fulfill your potential. The following is a list from Marilyn's book that beautifully captures what it means to be organized.[1] I've added examples related to healing in italics.

Being organized means:

> › You can find what you want when you need it, *like your medicine, exercise gear, cooking utensils, or supplements.*

> You can keep track of important information, *like your medical records, medical forms, health insurance records, recipes, or physical therapy instructions.*

> You can complete your tasks in a timely way, *creating less stress, more peace of mind, and more time to take care of your health.*

> You can arrive at your destination when you choose, *making all appointments more productive and less stressful.*

> You can take action when you want and seize new opportunities as they arise, *like a new treatment, diet, or exercise regime.*

> You can focus on what is important to you, *like exercise, researching treatments, preparing good food, more sleep, or time with friends and family.*

> You can do all this with a great degree of presence of mind, *which means decreased stress and increased joy, which we all know is good for your health.*

This list crystallizes how much a bit of order in your life can make a real difference. I say *a little bit of order* because, as with everything in this book, please remember that "a little bit is also good." We are seeking progress, not perfection. The goal is not to turn your closet into a Benetton display of perfectly folded clothes (mine certainly isn't). It is simply to insert a bit of order to help you heal.

>>> *For Today* <<<

Notice how you feel about this topic. Are you excited to get started, hopeless about getting more organized, resentful about being asked to explore it, or something else entirely? If you are feeling resistance, think about where that comes from, whether it is serving you in the long run, and how you might overcome it. You can also learn more about Marilyn's take on order and organizing at *www.MarilynPaul.com.*

)(

Day 92
Marilyn's Story: Know What's Important

*And now here is my secret, a very simple secret: It is only
with the heart that one can see rightly; what is essential is
invisible to the eye.*

—Antoine de Saint-Exupéry

Marilyn Paul, the author and organizing leader I mentioned in yesterday's entry, was married and had a 4-year-old son and a thriving consulting practice when she was diagnosed with stage 1 breast cancer. She was told she would need chemotherapy to shrink the large tumor her doctors found, and to follow the chemotherapy with surgery.

Like most individuals who learn that they have cancer, Marilyn said, "The shock was incredible." She continues:

Part of it was feeling a complete change in my life status. There was a shift in who I was. One day, I was walking around feeling fine, and the next day I was facing a life-threatening illness. But, there was something else that was kind of strange. That December was probably the best month of my adult life. My immediate response was, "Oh my God—I might not be here in a year." I was filled with joy and a new ability to savor every moment. I remember going to New York City for a few days and everything sparkled and the food tasted better. I felt so grateful.

Of course, later I thought, "Forget that!" and wasn't grateful for cancer at all. But, in those early moments, I really grasped viscerally our transience on this planet. Grasping that feeling helped me focus my organizing work later in my healing process.

What the diagnosis did was completely shift my understanding of what was important. I deeply understood that my life was limited and I realized what mattered—my health, being alive, celebrating life, being with my family, and taking good care of myself so I could do all that.

That shift in understanding enabled me to see that organizing isn't a matter of finding a better planner or being more disciplined; it's a matter of knowing what is important. What helps us manage our time and create order is not guessing or hoping we know what's important, but really viscerally knowing what is.

She continues: "As I went through chemo and surgery, it was hard for me to accept how little energy I had, but I finally grasped that the most important thing for me was to eat as well as I could and after that it was to spend time with my son, and then rest. That was it."

She also acknowledges that "to take care of myself well when I was that wiped out, with a young child, really required a major organizing effort." Here are a few organizing pieces that were key to supporting her healing:

> › Having a meeting early in the process with a few friends to discuss what help she needed, what she could ask for, and who might do what.

> › Keeping the kitchen organized and well-stocked so that making meals was easy for her or whoever was helping her.

> › Communicating clearly with lists and good instructions to anybody who was bringing meals, taking care of her son, or running an errand.

> › Delegating things to other people, like organizing meals or having someone come in to play with her son regularly.

> › Keeping the lines of communication clear with her husband so that they could work as a team to support her healing and their son's processing of the whole event.

"The hardest part was saying no to things and really letting myself rest," says Marilyn, "Resting was hard because I am such a doer. I found that having lots of order helped. I needed to feel held by simplicity. Having a pleasant, uncluttered space and eliminating all irrelevant e-mails made a big difference. I finally learned to rest deeply every day."[2]

»» *For Today* ««

What's most important to you? What are the clear priorities that you want to make time for and take care of in your healing work and the rest of your life?

><

Day 93
Organizing Is Holy, Healing Work

First a man should put his house together, then his town, then the world.

—Rabbi Yisroel Salanter

Creating order in your life so that you can take care of what really matters is holy work. In fact, in the Bible's original Hebrew, the word for "holy" is *kodesh*, which can also be translated as "set apart." Think about things that are designated as holy or *kodesh* in the Bible. The Sabbath is my favorite example of something "set apart"—in this case, a special time to connect with oneself, with other people, and with the Divine.

Creating order in our lives is setting apart that which really matters, and giving it the attention it requires. It removes impediments and enables us to become our most fully realized, authentic selves, and manifest the particular gifts and talents that nature and God gave us.

Applying a few organizing fixes like the following can make an enormous difference in your healing work and thus your ability to fully manifest your gifts in the world:

› Make one or two weekly menus with an associated grocery list so that you always have the ingredients you need to make nourishing, nurturing meals.

› Collect your medical records and lab results from healthcare providers and file them in a single notebook to help you take charge of your healthcare appointments and use them much more effectively.

› Bookmark Websites on your Internet search engine to clearly sort and tag any treatment that you may want to learn more about in the future.

Keep in mind that organizing fixes do not have to always be the obvious make-a-schedule or clean-out-a-drawer variety. Be creative and play to your strengths. Jeffrey, a 45-year-old human resources worker, was about 30 pounds overweight and had spent years trying to figure out how to get himself to watch less TV and exercise more. Finally he bought a used treadmill and put it in front of his TV. He lost the weight in six months. You never know what will make the difference.

>»> *For Today* «««
Choose one of the previous organizing fixes or another of your own and think about how you might make it happen, what gets in the way of doing it, and what support you could use to get past any obstacles?

)(

Day 94
Jump In: What's Your Relationship to Order?

Got up this morning and could not find my glasses. Finally had to seek assistance. Kate [Winslet] found them inside a flower arrangement.

—Emma Thompson

We all know people who seem naturally super-organized and others for whom making it to work each morning fully dressed and in possession of their keys, phone, and wallet is a struggle. As you already know, I lean toward the latter end of that spectrum.

For some people, a combination of an organized mind and the possession of good organizational habits (usually from childhood) makes creating order easy for them. For others, getting organized can be more challenging. This can be due to a range of things, including having gotten negative messages about housework or organizing as a young person, not having been taught helpful habits as a child, or, more significantly, having some form of ADHD or repercussions from a brain injury.

In Marilyn Paul's book, *It's Hard to Make a Difference When You Can't Find Your Keys,* she addresses many of those issues. According to Marilyn, our disorganization is just the tip of the iceberg, whereas the foundation of that iceberg is composed of deeply held beliefs.

Regardless of how challenging it is for you to get organized, working to adopt some of the skills, habits, and techniques described in the rest of this chapter can help make your healing work more effective. How each person interacts with this topic will look a little different. Explore the following questions to see what it all might mean for you.

1. Do you consider yourself to be a more organized or less organized person?

2a. *If you are more organized*: What are some ways that you are not applying your superior organizing habits to taking care of your health (in the same way that you might apply it to taking care of your finances, getting your job done, or cleaning your house)?

3a. Why do you think that you don't use all your organizing skills to help you take care of your health?

4a. How can you change that?

2b. *If you are less organized*: What beliefs about being organized might you hold that get in the way? Examples might be:[3]

• Modern women don't do housework.

• Cooking and housework is for women, not men.

• A clean desk is a sign of an empty mind.

• Clutter equals creativity.

• Neatness equals shallowness.

• Being overscheduled means you're important.

• I'm inherently disorganized and there is little I can do.

3b. How do those beliefs serve you now or get in your way?

4b. What can you do to change the beliefs that get in your way?

5b. What outside support can you get to help you overcome the beliefs and habits that get in your way (for example: work with an ADHD or executive function coach, have a session with a professional organizer, or get help from a more organized friend)?

✕

Day 95
Debbie's Story: Embrace Home-Care as Self-Care

*If you want to be healthy, you have to trade your wishbone
for a backbone and get to work.*

—Dr. Hazel Parcells

When I talk about bringing order into your home, I'm not talking about keeping it clean to impress company. I'm talking about putting time and attention into what is in your home and how it is organized, so that your belongings serve you in your efforts to get healthier, rather than get in the way. Debbie's story is a powerful illustration of how this can make a difference.

Debbie was 41 years old when she was suddenly debilitated by a back injury and transformed from an athletic business owner to an unemployed patient. Life as she knew it stopped. Lying down, sitting, or bending over caused searing pain to shoot through her chest and arms, so she spent endless days and nights standing or pacing, trying to control the pain.

Thus began a three-year odyssey through countless doctors' offices. As time passed, the pain spread throughout her body, to her muscles and joints, and she received a diagnosis of fibromyalgia, which essentially means "You're in pain and we don't know why." She could barely move and was on several pain medications to get through each day. Foot surgery during that time exacerbated the problem, leaving her with paralyzing pain running from her back to her head. "I was so full of drugs and in so much pain, I thought I was going to die," she says.

Finally, the key to Debbie's healing appeared in the unlikeliest of packages: skincare products. She received a gift from a friend from Beautycounter, a company that screens its products closely for possible toxins and bans 1,500 chemical substances of questionable safety. Debbie noticed that her skin was considerably healthier after using the new products for only a week.

She then began to research all the possibly toxic substances in her personal care and household products and food. Says Debbie:

> The most important decision I made to get healthy was to eat a diet free of processed foods, sugar, and any and all chemicals. Eventually, I removed all sugar, changed all foods in my

home to organic, increased our vegetable intake, got off all my medications, and changed all our products to toxin-free items. It wasn't easy. It took over a year to switch everything over and it is still a work in progress.

Slowly my health began to improve as I began to de-tox my body. I no longer have symptoms and am able to exercise like I used to before my initial back injury. What started out as an experiment with new facial products became a lifestyle change I would never have thought possible. It gave me back my life and I am so grateful.[4]

Add to Debbie's story the fact that 90 to 95 percent of cancers have their roots in environmental factors like smoking, diet, and toxins and radiation in our homes and workplaces.[5] That makes a compelling argument for using some organizing skills to declutter our homes, re-think our habits, and get rid of potentially toxic substances.

Fran Drescher, producer, actor, and writer known for the TV series *The Nanny* and *Happily Divorced*, is a uterine cancer survivor and the founder of the nonprofit Cancer Schmancer. Her campaign "Detox Your Home," provides materials and links at *www.CancerSchmancer.org* to help find safer products and share information with friends about creating a healthier home environment.

If you look into it a bit, it's crazy what's in some of our products. It's been in the news for a while that many lipsticks contain at least a trace of lead. Now, a new study has found that several lipstick brands contain as many as eight other metals, from cadmium to aluminum.[6] Similarly, popular glass cleaners tend to contain ammonium hydroxide and ethanolamine, both of which are toxic irritants that can contribute to respiratory ailments like asthma.[7]

We don't know the exact impact of all these substances on our bodies, but, at the very least, if you are trying to recover from a serious health condition, all those extra toxins aren't going to help. As Fran Drescher says, "I'm not going to wait for the government to tell me to stop eating strawberries soaked in pesticide and stop cleaning with potential carcinogens. We're not children. We can make our own decisions and lead the way. There's no harm in making the switch. Better safe than sorry!"[8]

One of the main reasons that people often give for not getting rid of potentially toxic products in their homes is that it is too much work. If you use the guidance from CancerSchmancer.org and some of the organizing principles described in this section on creating order, you can make it much easier.

>»> *For Today* «««
Find one or two products in your home that are going to need replacing soon and do some research on more natural alternatives. A great resource is *www.CancerSchmancer.org/check*.

)(

Day 96
Make Space for What Matters

Give me the discipline to get rid of the stuff that's not important, the freedom to savor the stuff that gives me joy, and the patience not to worry about the stuff that's messy but not hurting anybody.

—Vinita Hampton Wright

We just saw that one important element of embracing home care as self-care is being thoughtful about what is in your home and how it's being used. Decluttering is a great practice to help make that happen. Today, I want to share some decluttering gems from the FlyLady (*aka* Marla Cilley). Her Website, *www.FlyLady.net*, books, *Sink Reflections* and *Body Clutter*; and numerous organizing products are invaluable tools in learning how to make your home serve you instead of the other way around.

Shine Your Sink!

The FlyLady's first direction to her readers is "Shine your sink!" (I would add to do it with natural products.) Her theory is that a clean sink gives us the message that we are deserving of and capable of having a well-ordered, nurturing home. It can inspire us to keep the rest of the kitchen and the whole house in better order. This had a huge impact on my ability to heal. Shining my sink, and then making sure my sink and kitchen were clean every night, made it so much easier to make a green juice first thing every morning. And all those vitamin- and protein-packed juices played a major role in my healing.

You Can Do Anything for 15 Minutes

Setting a timer for 15 minutes and focusing intensely on getting as much filing, decluttering, or straightening done as possible can be a life-saver. Working in short chunks of time keeps you focused and won't wear you out. Plus, once you start decluttering for 15 minutes, you often find yourself continuing on longer, and after a few rounds have a whole new space to enjoy. I have met many people who were able to adopt a new self-care practice like yoga or weightlifting once they cleared boxes out of spare rooms or piles of papers out of their bedrooms to create an inviting space.

Put Out Your Hot Spots

There are surfaces in everyone's home that pile up with stuff on a regular basis. These hot spots are where sunglasses, single socks, parking tickets, and school forms go to die. My current hot spots are the kitchen counter by the back door, my nightstand, and the left side of my desk. The FlyLady encourages us to "put out" a hot spot or two by clearing things off it for even just a few minutes every day. That way, they won't get a chance to heat up the same way again.

Do a 27-Fling Boogie

Here is the FlyLady's description of this practice, straight from her Website at *www.flylady.net*: "Do this assignment as fast as you can. Take a garbage bag and walk through your home and throw away 27 items. Do not stop until you have collected all 27 items. Then close the garbage bag and pitch it. DO NOT LOOK IN IT! Just do it. Next, take an empty box and go through your home, collecting 27 items to give away..."[9] Add some music and this is one of my favorite activities.

Before we go further into this topic, I want to share one word of warning. I read recently that "Organizing is the new dieting." Just like improving your diet, organizing and decluttering can be immensely helpful. And, just like improving your diet, there are many pitfalls to avoid. If you find yourself doing any of the following, take note and recalibrate:

> › Organizing for appearance's sake, rather than to serve your own purposes.

> › Wasting energy feeling bad about yourself if you don't get "organized enough."

> › Overdoing an organizing project to avoid dealing with your health challenge.

> › Getting organized to an extreme and then feeling bad when it's not sustainable.

>>> *For Today* <<<

Grab a garbage bag and try a 27-Fling Boogie or set a timer for 15 minutes and take a whack at a hot spot. It feels so good.

ᐧ

Day 97
Set Up Your Space Like a Kindergarten Classroom

Simplicity is about subtracting the obvious and adding the meaningful.

—John Maeda

Though I had heard the phrase *a place for everything and everything in its place* a million times, I could never picture how that worked—that is, until Julie Morgenstern showed me how to set up my house like a kindergarten classroom in her fabulous book *Organizing From the Inside Out*.

A house organized like a kindergarten classroom doesn't mean that it's decorated in primary colors or overrun with stuffed animals. It's just well-organized. Julie calls this concept her "secret weapon" for organizing. Here is her description:

Walk into any kindergarten classroom in the world and you will behold the perfect model of organization. Think about what makes it work. First, the room is divided into activity zones: the Reading Zone, the Dress-up Zone, the Arts and Crafts Zone, the Music Zone and the Snack Zone.

Second...[e]ach zone is well-defined and fully self-contained, so that the child can concentrate 100 percent on a given task; nothing else competes for his or her attention.

Third, everything needed for each activity is right there at the child's fingertips because items are stored at their point of use. For example, if the child is doing arts and crafts, all the paper, crayons, markers, paints, brushes, and smocks needed for a creative session are gathered in one convenient location.

Fourth, in a kindergarten classroom it is almost as much fun putting things away as it is playing with them. Every item has a clear, well-labeled home in a container that is the perfect size to hold it.[10]

When I first read this description, two phrases jumped out at me. The first was *items are stored at their point of use*. For many people, including me, this can be revolutionary. For Joseph, a 50-year-old with sarcoidosis, an autoimmune disease that causes inflammation in various organs, putting all his yoga gear in one place made it possible to maintain a regular yoga practice. After years of struggling to commit to daily yoga, he realized that having his gear spread all over his apartment was getting in the way. His timer was in the kitchen; his yoga mat was shoved in the back corner of his bedroom closet; his yoga DVD was in a binder with music CDs in the living room; and his yoga block and strap were in a coat closet with the sports equipment. Just having to locate all that every morning was a major obstacle. Once he moved all the gear to an easily accessible spot near the living room where he liked to do yoga, he began doing it in the morning much more often.

The second phrase that struck me was *as much fun putting things away*. That has never been my experience. I hate cleaning up. I liked the idea that if everything were well-organized into categories and clearly labeled, cleaning up might actually be pleasant and my stuff would be easier to find.

Lisa is 35 and has rheumatoid arthritis. She tries hard to eat an anti-inflammatory diet recommended by her doctor. She works to increase her intake of vegetables and whole grains while avoiding refined carbohydrates, processed foods, and red meat. This has been a challenge for her and for her family. It became much easier and more pleasant for them all to make creative, healthy meals after she and her spouse and children spent a few hours decluttering, reorganizing, and labeling the kitchen and pantry shelves. Once they all knew where the ingredients and utensils were and could get them in and out easily—without causing an avalanche of Tupperware—they were all much more willing to get in the kitchen and see what they could do.

At this point your question might be "That's fine, but how do I do this? I'm not a kindergarten teacher or professional organizer." Agreed. Me neither. I spent one morning with a professional organizer to learn how. Tomorrow we'll explore the simple five-step technique to tame the chaos that I learned that morning.

>>>> *For Today* <<<<
Think about where in your home you might want to do some reorganizing to make your healthy habits more sustainable.

)(

Day 98
Five Steps to Organizing Your Space to Help You Heal

You can't organize clutter.

—The FlyLady

Laura Caufield, a wonderful professional organizer in the Boston area, showed up at my house at nine o'clock on a weekday morning ready to reorganize my children's basement play-space in four to six hours. I was amazed that she thought she could do it in that time. I had been putting it off for months because it looked like a multi-day job to me. But Laura was undaunted and we got it all done. Here are the five steps that I learned that day from working with Laura.

Step 1: Enlist Help
With Laura's help, I was able to organize the basement in a fraction of the time that it would have taken me otherwise. Her wisdom made a huge difference, but even just having a second mind and pair of hands helped a lot. Having support helps everybody get through tasks like this, but having it when you are sick or low energy can make it possible to get through the task at all. You may be able to do these jobs on your own, but it will be quicker, more pleasant, and more sustainable with help from family, friends, or a professional.

Step 2: Declutter

Here's a great rule of thumb. In order to allow an object to take up physical and energetic space in your home, it should be at least one of the following: very useful, very attractive, or very personally meaningful. If it is none of these, toss it. Set up three boxes or bags for garbage, recycling, and donations, and go to town freeing up your space and mind.

Step 3: Categorize

Once you have decluttered, it's time to categorize what is left. Make piles of things on floors or counters that are categorized according to their point of use—what they are used for and where they are used. All the art supplies go in one pile, whereas all the toy cars go in another. Often you can do steps 2 and 3 at the same time, tossing out and categorizing as you go.

Step 4: Put it All Away

Now, it's time to put everything in those piles away again; this time at their point of use. For example, put medications and supplements that are taken with meals in the kitchen, and pills that should be taken on an empty stomach in the bathroom.

Step 5: Label Everything

It's a real shame that most people skip this step. Labeling is what makes organizing sustainable. When you label things, you remember your new systems and other people can maintain your newly organized space for you. If you spend hours cleaning out your pantry and then your partner or roommate puts the groceries away in the old, random spots, it will be bad for your health in more ways than one. If your kitchen shelves have labels that say *snacks*, *juices*, *baking supplies*, and *cereal*, then that is what people will put there. If not, you'll have chaos again in two weeks. Try it. You may find buying an inexpensive label-maker and replacement tape to be one of the best purchases you ever make.

Congratulations! After you do these five steps, you will have a new, user-friendly space, which, with a little maintenance, will support your healthy living for months and years into the future. Again, this is not a must-do for every room of your house. Only do what makes a difference to you.

»»» *For Today* «««

Think of a space in your house that could use the kinder-garten-classroom treatment to make your health goals more attainable. Kitchens or bedroom closets are often good places to start. Ask a friend or family member to join you in the effort and set a date to dive in.

)(

Day 99
Create New Systems

Life is nothing without a little chaos to make it interesting.

—Amelia Atwater-Rhodes

Just like labeling in the decluttering process helps you maintain the order you create, developing systems in various areas of your life can help you return your belongings and spaces to order after they've been used. In *It's Hard to Make a Difference When You Can't Find Your Keys*, Marilyn Paul describes the "rhythm of organizing" like this: "...being organized is probably best described as a dynamic between a state of readiness for action and taking action. It is the rhythm of taking action, creating the natural disorder that comes with taking action, restoring order with helpful habits and useful systems, and thus returning to readiness for action."[11]

Here, I have applied Marilyn's stages of returning to order to making healthy meals in a clean kitchen:

Ready for Action = Kitchen with clear counters and sink and well-organized supplies.

Take Action = Prepare a healthy meal.

Natural Disorder = Kitchen gets messy.

Restore Order by Engaging Systems and Habits = Immediately wash all dishes and put away supplies.

Ready for Action = Orderly kitchen.

The challenge is that many of us don't have systems or habits that help us automatically move from the state of Natural Disorder to one of Ready for Action. We get stuck in that natural disorder for long periods in many areas of our life and it takes its toll, logistically, physically, and emotionally. Chaos is a natural part of life, but when we live there, our space and belongings are not Ready for Action, and neither are we.

In order to get back to Ready for Action, we need systems that automatically return us there. I highly recommend reading this section of Marilyn's book for more examples and a deeper explanation of how all this works. She explains that in order for systems that get you back to Ready for Action to work, they should play to your strengths, make sense to you, and be simple and low-maintenance. To get you started, here are two examples of simple systems that have worked for others.

Pillboxes: Buy some of the pillboxes with one container for each day. Schedule a time every Sunday when you organize your main medications and supplements into the boxes. This way you will always have your pills organized and know whether you have taken them or not. You can make it a pleasant weekly ritual with a healthy snack and some fun music.

Grocery list: Create a basic list on your computer that you pull out once each week and edit based on what's in your refrigerator and what you want to make the following week. Using an online grocery delivery service that saves your order from week to week online is immensely time-saving. This reduces stress, saves money, and helps ensure you always have healthy food to eat.

>>> *For Today* <<<
Choose one of the previously mentioned areas or another area of your life where you would like to have more order, and experiment with trying a new system.

)(

Day 100
Renovate Your Routines

*Routines are like mental butlers. Once you have a routine
in place, then the mental processes that make the behavior
happen take place automatically.*

—Michael McCullough

One of the most powerful ways to instill more order in your life is to renovate a routine. If you are having a hard time adopting a new self-care practice, completing a health-related task, or letting go of an unhealthy habit, creating a new routine that supports your health goals can make an enormous difference.

Here is an example of how I used a four-step process to create an evening routine that would enable me to get to bed earlier, get more higher quality sleep, and wake up early to exercise—all of which were key to my healing.

Step 1: Observe

A typical night went like this: I would read and cuddle with our two sons at their 8:30 p.m. bedtime. When I came out of their room at 9:00 or 9:30, I would be so exhausted that I couldn't face the kitchen-cleaning, e-mail-answering, and lunch-packing that needed to be done before I went to sleep. So, instead of just doing it and hopping in bed, I would "rest a bit" with some reading, TV, or Internet surfing. Bad idea. Before I knew it, it would be 10:00 p.m. and I wanted to do all that work even less. Finally, I would bring myself to do it all very slowly and fall into bed between 11:00 p.m. and 1:00 a.m.

Step 2: Analyze

Next, I identified what logistical obstacles were getting in the way of going to bed. The main things tripping me up were all the tasks I had to do before bedtime: answering e-mails, making lunches, and cleaning up the kitchen. By 9:00 p.m., I was just too tired to do those things efficiently. I needed to take those items off my plate at that hour so that I could be ready for bed as soon as my sons went to sleep.

Step 3: Strategize

After I identified what was causing the bedtime bottleneck, I needed to figure out how to move those to-do items off my plate at 9:00 p.m. First, I committed to not opening my e-mail account after 8:30 p.m. and taking 15 minutes to check e-mail each morning instead.

Second, I took up my husband, David, on an old offer to make lunches. I hadn't accepted originally because his lunches didn't seem as nutritious as mine. I got over that by giving him a list of suggested foods and recognizing that our sons would be better off with a well-rested mom than two more grams of fiber in their lunch boxes.

The last item I had to knock off my evening list was dinner cleanup on nights that David worked late and I was solo-parenting. I began focusing more on cleaning up as I cooked and made dinner earlier so that there was more time for cleanup. I also instituted a new rule that my sons (then 5 and 7) would help clean up for 10 minutes after every meal. Finally, I committed to staying in the kitchen after dinner until I had finished the entire cleanup by 7:30 or 8:00 p.m.

Step 4: Make the Change

Next, I had to implement all those changes and see if I could get in bed on time. Letting go of nighttime e-mail and handing over the lunch-making to David were fairly simple. But I had a much harder time sticking to my commitment to get the kitchen straightened up earlier. Part of the problem was that I felt that cooking was unimportant and didn't deserve much attention. So I would multitask my way through cooking—checking e-mail, talking on the phone, helping kids with their projects, and more—and wind up with a disaster area. Once I shifted my attitude and adopted a more focused, clean-up-as-you-go cooking style, the kitchen began to look less like a demolition zone after I finished.

Even after I had fine-tuned all of that, of course, it didn't always work. But most nights I was in bed by 9:30 p.m. and up by 6:00 a.m. It was a huge victory and a big step on my path to full health.

>>> *For Today* <<<

Choose one self-care practice that you have been having a hard time adopting. Follow the steps described here to begin to renovate your routines and make adopting that self-care practice more feasible. When looking at the obstacles, ask yourself: Exactly how does this get in my way? What are at least two ways that I could set up things differently? What support could I use to get past this obstacle? Routine renovations are unique to each person. Create the solutions that work best for you. As a gift to yourself, you can also go to *www.everydayhealingforyou.com/tools* and download for free "10 Recipes for a More Veggie-ful Life," which includes the main recipes that helped me get more vegetables into my life.

✕

»»»»»» Resources ««««««

I want to highlight these resources because they each helped change my life. Maybe they could help change yours, too. There are countless other books, health centers, blogs, and philosophies out there. Check these out, explore others, and find what works for you.

Practice 1: Take Charge

The Hippocrates Health Institute

Hippocrates offers revitalizing and detoxifying, live, plant-based food; treatments; education; and loving encouragement, all set in a beautiful campus in West Palm Beach, Florida. Visitors learn the ins and outs of a raw foods and green juice lifestyle here, including numerous detoxifying self-care practices.

Website: *www.hippocratesinst.org*

Kripalu

Kripalu is a yoga retreat center in Lenox, Massachusetts. Kripalu offers workshops and trainings in a number of yoga styles as well as multi-day programs led by national experts on a wide range of topics like Ayurvedic healing, discovering your inner artist, healing through song, and detoxifying cleanses.

Website: *www.kripalu.org*

Body Mind Restoration Retreats

These multi-day retreats are held at the Ithaca Zen Center in Ithaca, New York. They support healing through combining a live, plant-based diet and green juices with love, education, and meditation classes in a beautiful, restorative setting.

Website: *www.bodymindretreats.com*

Jack Canfield

Jack Canfield's book *The Success Principles* aims to help readers change how they approach life. It's full of great stories, tips, and advice for taking charge of your life and achieving your goals.

Website: *www.jackcanfield.com*

Alissa Cohen

Alissa Cohen's book, *Living on Live Food*, is a beautiful plant-based, living foods recipe book. Her inspirational stories and step-by-step instructions have helped so many people eat healthier by incorporating more fruits and vegetables into their diet.

Website: *www.alissacohen.com*

Jennifer Cornbleet

Jennifer Cornbleet's book, *Making Raw Food Easy for One or Two People*, is a must for anybody who wants to get more vegetables and protein-packed sprouts into their diet. Her recipes are simple, easy-to-follow, and made with ingredients and equipment that are readily available.

Website: *www.learnrawfood.com*

Colleen Patrick-Goudreau

Colleen Patrick-Goudreau's book, *The Vegan Table,* is chock-full of gorgeous pictures and delicious recipes. It is an excellent resource for people seeking to eat more vegetables.

Website: *www.joyfulvegan.com*

Practice 2: Nurture Your Heart

Martha Beck

Martha Beck's book, *The Joy Diet*: *10 Daily Practices for a Happier Life,* is a brilliant, funny primer on how to experience more joy and less anxiety. Covering topics like "Take Risks" and "Laugh More," she helps readers to create a more satisfying, joyful life.

Website: *www.marthabeck.com*

Gretchen Rubin

Gretchen Rubin's book *The Happiness Project* is a deep exploration of what makes us happy in every area of our life and why that matters. Her new book, *Better Than Before,* has some valuable insights on how we can start and keep new habits.

Website: *www.gretchenrubin.com*

Practice 3: Believe

The Benson-Henry Institute

The Benson-Henry Institute for Mind Body Medicine at Massachusetts General Hospital is a world leader in the study, advancement, and clinical practice of mind/body medicine. Their powerful in-person and online programs give participants a variety of mind/body skills to decrease medical symptoms and build confidence and resilience.

Website: *www.bensonhenryinstitute.org*

Practice 5: Create Order

Marilyn Paul

Marilyn Paul is a sought-after consultant and author of the best-selling book on getting organized *It's Hard to Make a Difference When You Can't Find Your Keys.* In addition to offering great organizing tips, her work helps people change how they think about organizing and thus overcome many blocks that make it difficult to take on new, healing habits.

Website: *www.marilynpaul.com*

Julie Morgenstern

Julie's books, *Getting Organized from the Inside Out* and *Time Management from the Inside Out,* help readers integrate more order into both their day and their belongings. From re-organizing a kitchen to make healthy cooking easier, to re-organizing a calendar to fit in daily exercise, Julie's wisdom can make healing work easier and more effective.

Website: *www.juliemorgenstern.com/books*

The FlyLady

The FlyLady (*aka* Marla Cilley) offers a system for organizing and managing one's life and home, based on daily routines and a focus on manageable tasks. Following her steps and adopting her mantras of "progress not perfection" and "I can do anything for 15 minutes" can help with the hard work of setting up a home to support healing.

Website: *www.flylady.net*

»»»»»» Notes ««««««

Introduction

1. Alan Morinis, *Every Day, Holy Day* (Boston: Trumpeter Books, 2010), 92.

Practice 1: Take Charge

1. Kay-Tee Khaw, et al, "Combined Impact of Health Behaviors and Mortality in Men and Women," *PLOS Medicine*, January 8, 2008. Accessed February 17, 2015, *http://journals.plos.org/plosmedicine/article?id=10.1371/journal.pmed.0050012.*
2. Martha E. Kilcoyne, *Defeat Chronic Fatigue Syndrome: You Don't Have to Live With It* (Sudbury, Mass.: Triple Spiral Press, 2007), 56–57.
3. Jennifer Gregg, et al, "Improving Diabetes Self-management Through Acceptance, Mindfulness, and Values," *Journal of Consulting and Clinical Psychology*, April 2007. Accessed February 17, 2015, *www.ncbi.nlm.nih.gov/pubmed/17469891.*
4. Marilyn Paul, *It's Hard to Make a Difference When You Can't Find Your Keys: The Seven-Step Path to Becoming Truly Organized* (New York: Viking, 2003). Exercise adapted from pp. 30–31.
5. Gretchen L. Zimmerman, et al, "A 'Stages of Change' Approach to Helping Patients Change Behavior," *American Family Physician*, March 2000. Accessed February 17, 2015, *www.aafp.org/afp/2000/0301/p1409.html.*
6. Suzanne C. Kobasa, et al, "Hardiness and Health: A Prospective Study," *Journal of Personality and Social Psychology*, January 1982. Accessed February 17, 2015, *http://dx.doi.org/10.1037/0022-3514.42.1.168.*
7. Some resources to learn more about *Mussar* include Alan Morinis's bestselling book, *Everyday Holiness* (Boston: Trumpeter Books, 2007), *www.mussarinstitute.org*, and *www.kirva.org.*
8. Rabbi Eliyahu Dessler, *Strive for Truth,* (Feldheim Publishers, 1978), 52–57.
9. Linda J. Vorvick (updated), "Exercise and Immunity," *Medline Plus,* updated May 15, 2012. Accessed February 17, 2015, *www.nlm.nih.gov/medlineplus/ency/article/007165.htm.*
10. Julie Corliss, "Too Much Sitting Linked to Heart Disease, Diabetes, Premature Death," *Harvard Health Blog*, January 22, 2015. Accessed February 18, 2015, *www.health.harvard.edu/blog/much-sitting-linked-heart-disease-diabetes-premature-death-201501227618.*

11. Diana Gerstacker, "Sitting is the New Smoking—7 Ways a Sedentary Lifestyle is Killing You," *The Active Times*, September 5, 2014. Accessed on February 18, 2015, *www.theactivetimes.com/sitting-new-smoking-7-ways-sedentary-lifestyle-killing-you?utm_source=huffington%2Bpost&utm_medium=partner&utm_campaign=sitting.*

12. Julie Corliss, "Too Much Sitting Linked to Heart Disease, Diabetes, Premature Death," *Harvard Health Blog.*

13. Bryan Walsh, "The Perils of Plastic," *Time*, April 1, 2010. Accessed February 18, 2015, *http://content.time.com/time/specials/packages/article/0,28804,1976909_1976908_1976938,00.html.*

14. Environmental Working Group, "Dirty Dozen Endocrine Disruptors," October 28, 2013. Accessed February 18, 2015, *www.ewg.org/research/dirty-dozen-list-endocrine-disruptors.*

15. All quotes are from personal interviews in December 2014.

16. If you want more brilliant advice from Ziesl Maayan or to learn about the integrated, holistic Functional Medicine approach that she and her colleagues use at Visions Medical Center in Dedham, Massachusetts, get in touch with them at *www.visionshealthcare.com.*

17. Ha T. Tu and Johanna Lauer, "Word of Mouth and Physician Referrals Still Drive Health Care Provider Choice," *Health System Change*, Research Brief No. 9, December 2008. Accessed February 18, 2015, *www.hschange.com/CONTENT/1028/.*

18. "Impact of Communication in Healthcare," *Institute for Healthcare Communication,* July 2011. Accessed February 18, 2015, *http://healthcarecomm.org/about-us/impact-of-communication-in-healthcare/.*

19. Marie Savard, "Doctor's Appointment? Don't Go It Alone," *ABC News,* July 28, 2008. Accessed February 18, 2015, *http://abcnews.go.com/Health/story?id=5452295.*

20. Hardeep Singh, "The Battle Against Misdiagnosis," *Wall Street Journal*, August 7, 2014. Accessed February 18, 2015, *www.wsj.com/articles/hardeep-singh-the-battle-against-misdiagnosis-1407453373.*

21. Stephen R. Covey, *The 7 Habits of Highly Effective People* (New York: Simon & Schuster, 1989).

Practice 2: Nurture Your Heart

1. Mayo Clinic Staff, "Stress Relief from Laughter? It's No Joke," Mayo Clinic Website. Accessed February 18, 2015, *www.mayoclinic.org/healthy-living/stress-management/in-depth/stress-relief/art-20044456.*

2. Judith Orloff, "The Health Benefits of Tears," *Psychology Today,* July 27, 2010. Accessed February 18, 2015, *www.psychologytoday.com/blog/emotional-freedom/201007/the-health-benefits-tears.*

3. Thich Nhat Hanh, "How to Practice Compassionate Listening," *Awaken Teachers*, August 31, 2014. Accessed February 18, 2015, *www.awaken. com/2014/08/thich-nhat-hanh-how-to-practice-compassionate-listening/*.

4. All quotes are from personal interviews in January 2015.

5. Zach Johnson, "Oprah Winfrey Ponders the Power of Gratitude," *E! Online*, October 8, 2014. Accessed February 18, 2015, *www.eonline.com/ news/586568/oprah-winfrey-ponders-the-power-of-gratitude*.

6. Amy Morin, "7 Scientifically Proven Benefits Of Gratitude That Will Motivate You To Give Thanks Year-Round," *Forbes*, November 23, 2014. Accessed February 18, 2015, *www.forbes.com/sites/ amymorin/2014/11/23/7-scientifically-proven-benefits-of-gratitude-that-will-motivate-you-to-give-thanks-year-round/*.

7. Martha Beck, "The Joy Diet: A Brief Guide to Feasting on Life," Martha Beck Website, May 1, 2003. Accessed February 18, 2015, *http:// marthabeck.com/2003/05/the-joy-diet/*.

8. R. Robinson, D.N. Khansari, A.J. Murgo, and R.E. Faith, "How Laughter Affects Your Health: Effects of Stress on the Immune System," *Immunology Today* 11, no. 5 (1990), 170–75.

9. Elise Craig, "When Doctors Need Doctors: Beating Breast Cancer with Help from Beyoncé," *San Francisco* magazine, December 18, 2014. Accessed February 18, 2015, *www.modernluxury.com/san-francisco/story/ when-doctors-need-doctors-beating-breast-cancer-help-beyonce*.

10. Martha Beck, "The Joy Diet: A Brief Guide to Feasting on Life."

11. Gretchen Rubin, "Why Samuel Johnson is the Patron Saint of My Happiness Project," *The School of Life* Website, May 18, 2011. Accessed February 18, 2015, *http://theschooloflife.typepad.com/the_school_of_ life/2011/05/gretchen-rubin-why-samuel-johnson-is-the-patron-saint-of-my-happiness-project.html*.

12. From a personal interview in January 2015.

13. Lissa Rankin, *Mind Over Medicine: Scientific Proof That You Can Heal Yourself* (Carlsbad, Calif.: Hay House, 2013), Chapter Four.

14. Ibid.

15. Ibid.

16. Courtney Spradlin, "Ill Woman's Living Wake Becomes Surprise Wedding," *USA Today*, December 23, 2014. Accessed February 18, 2015, *www.usatoday.com/story/news/nation/2014/12/23/living-wake-terminal-cancer-becomes-surprise-wedding/20798623/*.

17. Ibid.

Practice 3: Believe

1. Kendra Cherry, "Benefits of Positive Thinking," *About.com*. Accessed February 18, 2015, *http://psychology.about.com/od/PositivePsychology/a/ benefits-of-positive-thinking.htm*.

2. Lissa Rankin, *Mind Over Medicine: Scientific Proof That You Can Heal Yourself,* Chapter One.

3. Quotes and information from Professor Ted J. Kaptchuk are from a personal interview on March 2, 2015.

4. Rebecca Erwin Wells and Ted J. Kaptchuk, "To Tell the Truth, the Whole Truth, May Do Patients Harm: The Problem of the Nocebo Effect for Informed Consent," *The American Journal of Bioethics*, 12(3): 22–29, 2012.

5. Julie Steenhuysen, "Optimists Live Longer and Healthier Lives: Study," *Reuters*, March 5, 2009. Accessed February 18, 2015, *www.reuters.com/ article/2009/03/05/us-optimist-health-idUSTRE5247NO20090305.*

6. Elizabeth Scott, "The Benefits of Optimism," *About.com*, December 16, 2014. Accessed February 18, 2015, *http://stress.about.com/od/ optimismspirituality/a/optimismbenefit.htm*.

7. All quotes are from personal interviews in December 2014.

8. This story is attributed to the Chofetz Chaim, a leading European rabbi and scholar in the late 19th and early 20th centuries. This version is abridged and adapted from *Everyday Holiness* by Alan Morinis.

9. Rachel Eddins, "Working with Your Inner Critic," *Psych Central*. Accessed February 18, 2015, *http://psychcentral.com/lib/working-with-your-inner-critic/00017552*.

10. Mayo Clinic Staff, "Chronic Stress Puts Your Health at Risk," Mayo Clinic Website Accessed February 18, 2015, *www.mayoclinic.org/healthy-living/stress-management/in-depth/stress/art-20046037.*

11. Department of Health and Human Services and Centers for Disease Control and Prevention, *Exposure to Stress.* Accessed February 18, 2015, *www.cdc.gov/niosh/docs/2008-136/pdfs/2008-136.pdf.*

12. Susan Krauss Whitbourne, "The Six Best-kept Secrets About Stress," *Psychology Today*, March 12, 2013. Accessed February 18, 2015, *www. psychologytoday.com/blog/fulfillment-any-age/201303/the-six-best-kept-secrets-about-stress*.

13. Ashutosh Sharma, "How You Perceive Stress Matters," *Talk It Out!* Website, April 21, 2014. Accessed February 18, 2015, *https:// cucumbermanagement.wordpress.com/2014/04/21/how-you-perceive-stress-matters/*.

14. Ibid.

15. Herbert Benson, et al (1974), "The relaxation response," *Psychiatry* 37(1): 37–46. Analyzes the central nervous system response underlying the altered state of consciousness known as the relaxation response. The physiological states which appear to be operating are described, as well as techniques for inducing the response. Eastern and Judeo-Christian writings which describe the relaxation response are cited. Recent

practices are analyzed, including autogenic training, hypnosis, Zen, yoga, and transcendental meditation. Possible therapeutic benefits are discussed. (63 ref) (PsycINFO Database Record (c) 2012 APA, all rights reserved.) National Center for Complementary and Integrative Health.

16. "Meditation: What You Need to Know," NIH Website. Accessed February 18, 2015, *https://nccih.nih.gov/health/meditation/overview.htm*.

17. To purchase, visit *www.bensonhenryinstitute.org/13-store-resources/138-buy-our-meditation-recordings-on-itunes* and download free at *http://marc.ucla.edu/body.cfm?id=22*. Accessed February 18, 2015.

18. "Preparing for the End of Life," NIH Senior Health Website. Accessed February 18, 2015, *http://nihseniorhealth.gov/endoflife/preparingfortheendoflife/01.html*.

19. Haruki Murakami, *Blind Willow, Sleeping Woman: Twenty-four Stories* (New York: Knopf, 2006).

20. "Crazy Sexy Cancer's Kris Carr," Super Soul Sunday, Oprah Winfrey Network, November 10, 2013. Accessed February 18, 2015, *www.youtube.com/watch?v=k5cE3OnOZR4*.

21. "An Update on Crazy Sexy Cancer's Kris Carr," Super Soul Sunday, Oprah Winfrey Network, November 8, 2013. Accessed February 18, 2015, *www.youtube.com/watch?v=8rMoQesq05Y*.

22. "Crazy Sexy Cancer's Kris Carr," Super Soul Sunday, Oprah Winfrey Network, November 10, 2013.

23. Ibid.

Practice 4: Connect

1. Bert N. Uchino, et al, "The Relationship Between Social Support and Physiological Processes: A Review With Emphasis on Underlying Mechanisms and Implications for Health," *Psychological Review*, 1996. Accessed February 18, 2015, *http://psych.utah.edu/people/people/uchino/Publications/1996%20Uchino%20PB.pdf*.

2. Lisa F. Berkman, et al, "Emotional Support and Survival After Myocardial Infarction," *Annals of Internal Medicine*, December 15, 1992. Accessed February 18, 2015, *http://annals.org/article.aspx?articleid=706000*.

3. Tara Parker Pope, "Married Cancer Patients Live Longer," *New York Times*, September 24, 2013.

4. Danielle Ofri, "When the Patient is Non-Compliant," *New York Times*, December 15, 2012.

Practice 5: Create Order

1. Marilyn Paul, *It's Hard to Make a Difference When You Can't Find Your Keys: The Seven-Step Path to Becoming Truly Organized* (New York: Viking, 2003), 9.

2. All quotes in this profile come from a December 4, 2014 personal interview.

3. These examples are adopted from similar ones on pages 63–64 of *It's Hard to Make a Difference When You Can't Find Your Keys*.

4. All quotes in this profile come from a November 2014 personal interview.

5. Preetha Anand, et al, "Cancer is a Preventable Disease that Requires Major Lifestyle Changes," *Pharmaceutical Research*, September 2008. Accessed February 18, 2015, *www.ncbi.nlm.nih.gov/pmc/articles/PMC2515569/*.

6. Deborah Blum, "Is There Danger Lurking in Your Lipstick?" *New York Times*, August 16, 2013. Accessed February 18, 2015, *http://well.blogs. nytimes.com/2013/08/16/is-there-danger-lurking-in-your-lipstick/?_r=0*.

7. "EWG's Guide to Healthy Cleaning," Environmental Working Group Website. Accessed February 18, 2015, *www.ewg.org/guides/cleaners/1418-WindexAdvancedGlassMultiSurfaceCleaner*.

8. From a January 26, 2014 personal interview.

9. Accessed February 18, 2015, *www.flylady.net*.

10. Julie Morgenstern, *Organizing from the Inside Out* (New York: Henry Holt and Company, 1998), 50.

11. *It's Hard to Make a Difference When You Can't Find Your Keys*, 96.

Index

A

Acceptance and Commitment Therapy (ACT), 33

Acceptance, 31-38

Action, 45-46

Actions, feelings and, 77-78

Addictions, 119-120

Ambition, 40

Appointment buddy, 67, 160-161

Asking for help, 147-155, 173-185

Assumptions, 60-61

B

Baim, Peg, 107

Beck, Martha, 93-95, 97

Benson, Dr. Herbert, 130

Breath, power of, 133

Burden, 148

C

Cancer – 24, 30-31, 38, 40, 53-54, 90-92, 96, 100, 103, 112, 115, 124, 128, 143-144, 146, 169-170, 181, 190-191, 196-197

Cancer treatment, support for recovery from, 169-171

Carr, Kris, 143-145

Caufield, Laura, 201

Cerebral palsy, 97-98

Change Model, Stage of, 45-47

Childcare, outsourcing, 163

Choices, 51-53

Chronic Fatigue Syndrome, 15, 18-20, 31-33, 43, 108, 128, 167, 176-177, 179

Chronic Lyme Disease, 15, 18-20, 62, 124, 167, 179

Chronic pain, 16, 24, 27-29, 40-42, 55, 57-59, 64, 14, 16, 13, 176, 195-195

Cilley, Marla, 197-199

Cohan, Dr. Deborah, 96

Cohen, Alissa, 135

Commitment, 33, 47-51

Contemplation, 45-46

Covey, Stephen, 39, 71-72

Creating order, 187-206

Crum, Alia, 126

Crying, 82-86

Curiosity, 59-61

D

Death, 139-143

Decluttering, 196 – 203

Deep listening, 88-90

Denial, 31-36

Dessler, Rabbi Eliyahu, 52

Destination, Inspiring, 39-42

Diabetes, 24, 31, 33, 41-42, 53-56, 97, 126, 149-150, 176

Diet, 54-56

Drescher, Fran, 196-197

E

Eating habits, 54-56

Eddins, Rachel, 119-120

Eldercare, outsourcing, 164

Embracing change, 42-43

Emotional obstacles, 75-80

End of life, 139-143

Errands, outsourcing, 162

Expectations, 39, 66

Experimentation, 23-24

Exposure to toxins, 54, 195-197

F

Fear, 17, 75, 80-81

Feasting, 93-94

Feedback, 113-114

Feelings, 75-84

Fibromyalgia, 176, 195-196

Fight-or-flight response, 124-125

Finding a physician, 62-65

FlyLady, 197-199

Functional Medicine, 60

G

Gerzon, Robert, 123

God, 24-25, 50-51, 114-116, 148, 155

Gratitude, 93, 132

H

Hand in Hand Parenting, 84

Healing cycle, 23-24

Healthcare team, 56-57

Heart, nurturing your, 75-101

Heart disease, 31, 53, 104, 108, 128

Help, asking for, 147 -155, 173-185

Help, healing and, 146-149

Hopelessness, 29-31

Housework, outsourcing, 162-163

Hyman, Dr. Mark, 60

I

Information, managing, 68-70

Inner critic, 118-124

Inspiration, 40

Inspiring Destination, 39-42

Irritable Bowel Disease, 57-59

Isolation, 145, 155

J

Journal, 22

Joy, 93-101

K

Kaptchuk, Ted J., 106, 107

Kilcoyne, Martha E., 31-33

L

Labeling, 202

Laughter, 82-84, 95

Lessons, learning, 37-39

Life, end of, 139-143

Limits, 50-51

Listening partnerships, 82-92

Listening, deep, 88

Logistical obstacles, 75-76

M

Maintenance, 24, 45 46

Mammalian brain, 80-81, 84

Managing information, 68-70

Meal preparation, outsourcing, 163

Medicine, Functional, 60

Money, 164-166

Mood, 104

Morgenstern, Julie, 199

Morinis, Alan, 23

Multiple Sclerosis, 24, 55, 61, 176

Mussar, 23, 51-53, 115-116

N

Negativity, 117-124

Neocortex, 80-81

Nocebo effect, 106-107

O

Obstacles, emotional, 75-80

Obstacles, logistical, 75-76

Ofri, Dr. Danielle, 149

Optimism, 107-113

Order, 17, 142, 187-206

Organization, 187-206

Outcomes, 40

Outsourcing, 162-164

P

Parkinson's Disease 24, 46, 62

Partnerships, listening, 82-92

Passion, 22-23

Patience, 22-23

Patient Health Questionnaire, 94

Patterns, 87

Paul, Marilyn, 34, 188-191, 193, 203-204

Perception, 125

Perfection, progress vs., 21, 172, 189

Persistence, 46-46, 156

Physician, Communication with, 63

Physician, finding a, 62-65

Placebo effect, 105-107

Plant-based diet, 15, 20, 55, 144, 151

Positive outlook, 103-105

Positivity, 40, 117-124

Pre-contemplation, 45-46

Preparation, 45-46

Primary support person, 156-159

Prioritization, 128-129

Progress, perfection vs., 21, 172, 189

Q

Questioning assumptions, 60-61

R

Rankin, Dr. Lissa, 98-99, 105

Relapse, 45-47

Relationships, deepening, 146-147

Relaxation response, 130-133

Reptilian brain, 80-81, 84

Research, 23, 59-61

Resignation, 37

Responsibility, 16, 27, 66

Role model, 166-168

Rothfeld, Dr. Glenn, 112

Routines, 203-206

Rubin, Gretchen, 97

S

Self-worth, 173-176

Sitting, 53-54

Stages of Change Model, 45-47

Stress, 124-129

Suffering, 34-38

Support person, primary, 156-159

Support system, 17, 34, 145-185

T

Team, healthcare, 56-57

Time management, 71-73

Toxins, exposure to, 54, 195-197

Traumatic brain injury, 109-111

Trust, 114-116

Truth, 31-33

V

Visualization, 133-137

W

Weight loss, support for, 170-171

Whitbourne, Dr. Susan Krauss, 126

Janette Hillis-Jaffe combines her personal experience as a patient with her background as a public health professional to help others chart a course out of illness into health. Janette is a sought-after speaker, consultant, and coach, with a master's in public health from the Harvard School of Public Health. She spent thousands of hours studying counseling, nutrition, the mind-body connection, and the U.S. healthcare system during her successful effort to heal from her own six-year debilitating autoimmune disorder. Having recovered her health, she lives in Sharon, Massachusetts, and supports others to lose weight, ease chronic illness, recover from acute illness, and overcome persistent pain. For more information, please go to *www.healforrealnow.com*.